Lose Weight

With A

Smile

Lose Weight

With A

Smile

S.R.SHUJA

First Edition

Cover page: Zakeem Shuja

Printed in the United States of America

Publisher: Mind Talkers Publishing
Ajax, Ontario, Canada

ISBN #:978-0-9878187-7-5

Visit www.mindtalkers.com

To good health and happiness

Table of Content

Prologue

Losing weight is not easy. To some it may even seem impossible. However, in this time of increasing obesity among general population – adult and children both - it is one thing that is becoming popular albeit slowly. Considering the fact that under normal circumstances a fit body undisputedly represents better health and higher energy level, keeping ones weight within reasonable limits can only have better outcome. No wonder, plenty of people have figured this simple truth out and are trying their best to get in shape. However, this is probably one area where trying and achieving could be completely two different things. That's where I come. Like many others out there I'll attempt to help my readers to get the best out of their effort by sharing the knowledge that I have gained from my own experience over the years.

I was really skinny in my childhood. I had gained some weight during my youth but was still very lean, totally devoid of any discernible fat. However, like everything else, my body changed over time as well. During a patch of depression, slightly aimless and disappointed, I started to fancy on foods. It did not take very long before none of my cloths fit me anymore. Very soon I became slightly overweight to heavily overweight. With my trouser buttons refusing to co-operate I soon became totally dependent on the belt to save my decency.

Then, one fine morning, I realized what I had to do. There was no excuse, no escaping the truth. *I did not like the way I looked. I did not like the way I felt. I did not like the way others reacted with my size and appearance.*

It was time to bounce back.

It took me months after months of hard work, hundreds of hours of studies, many cumbersome experiments with food, exercise, medicines - what not. I lost some; gained back some; got frustrated, quit only to collect myself again and dive back in the cyclic process. Lose, gain, give up; lose, gain, give up... Eventually I have figured out a way that not only works but works without putting me through unnecessary stress. Now, not only I know how to keep myself fit and healthy, I can actually make myself feel great while doing so.

So, here I am, writing a book on losing weight. Or is it really about losing weight? Never for a moment have I thought that weight loss alone can become a motivating factor to carry a person through the hardship that comes with it. If such activities do not help us feel better and happier then what good would it do? If you ask me, losing weight is really about being fit, being healthy and being happy. That's why my book is titled **'Losing weight with a smile'**. Note dear readers, I do not promise that you can go on eating that calorie packed cheese cake and still somehow follow my method to lose weight. I simply do not have any magical formula. Neither do I want to hide behind cleverly crafted wordings and fine prints. I'll get to things in a straight forward, matter of fact way. You'll have to adapt to it. It works for me. It'll work for you too. Have confidence in me.

I'll reinforce on the first statement that I made – **losing weight is not easy**. In fact it is difficult and often tough. It may hurt in all areas – body, mind, finance, comfort. It is a given fact that most people who attempt it either totally fails and simply gives up or succeeds partially only to relapse back to the beginning. Only a handful succeeds in the long term. No, I am not going to promise success. I have already mentioned that I am not a magician. I cannot make you do anything unless you are determined to do so. Promising you something that I cannot deliver is not the reason why I started this effort. My goal is to give you hope. Assist you with your noble attempt and provide you with some positive and proven directions to succeed. Anyway, that's enough of babbling. Are you ready to do this? While this book may look small in size the actual impact of it should be strong enough to stay for years. This is definitely not a book that you plan to read once and put aside to be forgotten. It is expected to become a friend and companion as you continue in your journey to get in shape. Keep it handy. Follow my directions – loosely or strictly, whatever suits you. Good luck.

Chapter 1

Why?

Why should you lose weight?

Even before you can shed an ounce you need to ask yourself this universal question.

Why should I lose weight?

Or putting it slightly differently: why anyone would even be crazy enough to step into a life style of painful dieting, exercising and all the other inconveniences that comes with it. Most of us know how easy it is to gain weight − a little overeating, slight lack of physical activities, a few parties and suddenly all these unwanted fat and flesh gathers in abundance primarily into the regions we hate them the most - belly, legs, butt; at least that's how it feels like. The truth may be far apart from that but it inevitably feels like that. When did it happen? How could I let myself slip to this? All kind of questions pops up in the mind.

Let's forget for a moment how it happened. Let's focus on the fact that we have set up our mind to get rid of the extra weight. But before going ahead we need to know a clear answer to the question – **Why**? It is an important question. Actually it is the most important question in this journey. You must have noticed my choice of word – *journey*. It truly is a journey and that is why you must know whether you have the right reasons to embrace this journey.

It is easy to realize that the answer to that question will be different for different people – though not so different that they cannot be categorized. I am going to lay out the categories and let you determine where you fall. If I have missed any please feel free to add it.

- Health issues
- Peer pressure
- Family pressure
- Self realization
- Uncomfortable with existing appearance
- Psychological problems
- Other [Yours to add]

I must insist that you do this first. Don't allow yourself

to get snobby. If you have decided to walk with me please play by my rule. At the end it's you who'll benefit. Like physical laws everything runs on some basic principles. It is essential to learn those principles. The time will come when you won't need me trying to mentor you. But for now, let's go slow, one step at a time.

In your quest to determine the answer to '**Why**' I suggest you talk to yourself. It is a better idea to do so in a place where nobody else is present so that they don't start wondering about the state of your mind. It has a hypnotic effect on human mind. If you know the answer to '**why**' that's a good start. If you are not very clear about it or do not feel as strongly as you want to then use the '*talk to yourself*' method. Stand before a mirror and tell yourself what you want from you. We all have at least two personalities – one the doer, the other is the reviewer. Let the reviewer take the driving seat, let it guide the doer. All these might sound like weird psychological stuff but it works.

Okay, let's move on. Let's assume that you have done whatever is necessary and have a clear understanding and possibly an answer to the nagging '**why**' question.

I don't know what your answer is but I can't pass on the opportunity to make a wild guess - *you want to fit inside your favorite dress that you couldn't wear for last five summers.* If you are a man then – I don't know – *maybe you are thinking of starting to look like me – all fit and athletic, happy and cheerful, enjoying the interested look from all those pretty, youthful women.* Okay, that was quite a bit of exaggeration but you get the idea. I do get some nice furtive looks every now and then from desperate middle aged women, but who can blame them!

How to build <u>Motivation</u>

Just knowing the answer to 'why' can't possibly do any good if we cannot use that answer in our advantage to create a good load of motivation – the most important factor in all these weight loss activities.

Being healthy is really what we should be seeking for – ideally. One might wonder whether big can be healthy. The answer may be tricky. In the short term many overweight athletes may show great skill and fitness but over time what would evidently become important is being proportionately sized. There are several units that are used to determine such appropriateness like height to weight ratio, BMI (Body Mass Index) etc. Generally speaking any unnecessary accumulation of flesh and fat are bound to do some harm, not always quickly but usually steadily. And of course there is that factor of being the subject of ridicule which no matter how strong minded one might be is bound to be the cause of plenty of grief.

Again I insist that before you move on you come up with a good *motivation*, one or more if you are lucky, and plant it clearly and strongly in your mind. Without a solid and long living motivation this venture not going anywhere, I can say that to you with confidence. Make no mistake by *motivation* I do not ask you to come up with a major plan about your goals and target of life. Just having one or more loosely understood reasons or causes to create some continuous drive to stay in the program is all you need. *Continuous* is the word of the day here.

What is my motivation? Simple. I really enjoy looking shapely. It gives me intense pleasure to show off my lanky outlook in a world where most middle aged men either looks bulky or overweight and withdrawn with a balding head which I so delightfully share. Delightfully because this balding thing have scored big with my young kids and I love to share laughter with them when they come up with funny things to say. Anyway, the sportive attitude and energy provides me a kick that is truly enjoyable. It provides me a very good reason to continue into the next day and the day after that. It's all good news. I want the same for you. If you are already there, happiness and satisfaction wise, great, I'll make it stay longer.

Okay, enough of harassment. You must be bored to death by now wondering if I would ever get out of this worthless *'why'* and *'motivation'* cycle. I stop right here. Let's just assume you are determined, so determined that not even the mighty Himalaya can change your mind. Admitted, that was a poor statement but you get the idea. Let's get into business.

Chapter 2

How?

How to lose weight?

I am sure you have already done some research of your own and are already aware of few things about losing weight. You must have also seen the so familiar weight loss ads promising sure solutions to become a beautiful well shaped model, male or female. All you have to do is to follow their system. These businesses tout all kind of stuff — from miracle no stress diet to miracle drugs — promising weight loss without the hardship. Do they actually work? Don't ask me. I am one of those unfortunates who simply do not believe in miracles. Everything happens as a result of subsequent events or efforts, often remaining out of our knowledge. I am not claiming to know the truth about all miracle solutions. You are free to try. I don't necessarily discount them. However, I do not advice making them your sole approach to a difficult problem, just in case you decide to give them a try. However, I must also caution about taking dubious medicines or similar stuff. Possibly a good idea would be to speak to a doctor of medicine before putting any of those into your system.

Okay, now the million dollar question. How to get rid of the unwanted weight? The answer is simple - **by hard work** and **methodical approach**. Four important elements are: **motivation**, **dieting**, **work out** and a **solid strategy**. Some of you probably already hate all or some of them. But don't get alarmed. That's where I come in. My primary goal is not just to show you a way but also to try to make it easier for you to follow. I pay a lot of attention to strategy, even to things that are apparently very well known. A good strategy should have two simple parts. First part is *where we ask the questions*. In the second part *we try to find a procedure to answer the questions*. What can be some of the possible questions? How? What? When?

I know you must have already tried several approaches, at least partially. Some might have worked, some might not. Not to worry. You are in good hands. I am not just going to take the role of adviser. I'll be your trainer, companion and a trusted friend. Everything I'll tell you are things that I have applied successfully several times on me and hopefully will be able to help you all the way to fitness and prosperity. Before we start it is important to discuss about some important things.

Why are there so many <u>systems</u>?

If one system in one singular form worked for everybody then there would have been no need for other options. Unfortunately that is never the case. Different processes work better for different set of people based on their life styles, preferences and often cultural views. Multiple systems invariably pop up in areas where there is interest in alternatives. Weight loss is an area where generally common acceptable approaches are based on hard work and difficult practices. As a result many do seek out for relatively easier approaches. There is nothing wrong about that. Following a combination of approaches may not always be a bad idea provided they do not have opposing views. But as the wise men say – if something sounds too good to be true then it is very likely not true. Not all systems work. Not all systems can even be considered as systems. Some are just shameless effort to cater ineffective materials to desperate people who are eager to hold on to straws.

It's all about business – obviously!

Can I experiment?

You may but do you really want to? Or do you need to? I am writing this book based on my experiences and experiments over the years as I tried to find a good, reasonably stable approach that works. While you are free to do your own experiments my suggestion would be to not waste energy and time in such activities and simply follow this proven procedure. However, if you do decide to experiment, remember not to go for random approaches and not to mix up drastically different ones. By doing so you would not be able to measure correctly which one worked to what extent if they really did. Unplanned experiments usually cannot sustain over time. It is better to pick a system, study it, analyze it and follow it to determine if it is suitable to your needs. For long term result it is important to pick a system that is most effective to you.

Why not take what worked for me?

If you ask for my advice, I would ask you not to experiment. At least for the first full scale effort try a method that has already been tested. There are too many systems out there, you may get lost if try to check every one of them.

I have done the homework

Do yourself a favor – clear your mind and stay with me. At the end you'll find a system that is easy to follow and works without failure. I have been successfully maintaining for over fifteen years now. You'll also be able to do so and be happy about it.

Be assured I am going to do more than just sharing my experience. I am actually going to teach you, guide you and often may even be insisting on you. All of these are good for you. I am going to be your coach, friend and mentor, if you allow me to be. However, for that relationship to succeed you must take my words in your heart and follow my advice and instructions.

Since I started my quest to lose weight and get to a point where I can be comfortable with my body I have gone in several directions. None of them were easy. But I didn't mind because I always believed in reasonable hard work without losing my mind and happiness. Honestly speaking, that is not always possible if you are too materialistic. It is a state of mind, a way of thinking without losing your own ways. But before we start lets set up a few rules for ourselves:

Lose weight, not happiness.

Not happy with your body? Work hard until satisfied.

No worries about occasional lapses.

Occasional lapses must not lead to large scale collapses.

Smile throughout the process (as the title demands).

Let's do something important for the rest of our lives...

Chapter 3

Objective

Where you are?

First question first: What is your current condition? Do you consider yourself fat... very fat... not so fat...

What do you mean by fat?

I apologize if I have in anyway offended you by using the word *fat* but often being able to call yourself *fat* (if you are overweight) is really the first step toward redemption. Please do not misunderstand me. If you are still with me that means you are really desperate and have some kind of belief that I can help you to get there. And it is my personal opinion that being able to define something is important. If you want to keep your motivation going it is far better to think of a slightly funny and may be a little humiliating word than something that almost make it sound honorable – overweight. Almost like middleweight, heavyweight etc. Do yourself a favor, if you are overweight call yourself fat. The worse you feel the better. Remember there's nothing to smile about being unhealthy, obese, overweight and simply fat.

I'll ask the question again.

What is your current condition?

Take a copybook, write it down. Write down your weight, exact condition and time of measurement. This reference will play a good role in future. However, the goal is never to just sail down the line from there. A lot may happen since you start. But this information needs to stay intact. A good reference point works very well for motivation. Do not forget your target may actually change for better or worse, that is part of flexibility, to ensure long term sustainability.

Where you want to be?

Okay, finally we have come to the point where you must decide exactly what you want from this exercise? You want to lose weight, I get that. However, it is now necessary to determine how much weight you want to lose. Also, do you have any particular requirement on where the weight needs to be reduced? It is quite possible that your requirements cannot be met but it is still very good to identify and list.

How far you think you want to go?

Ask yourself once more: is your target too high? Can you reasonably reach there in a specific time period? It is important to remember that while there are some cases with extreme success – be it short term or long term, the truth is for most people the success either is very short living or never really comes. Hence setting up a pretty big target will serve no good. Instead it's better to setup a target for next six months which may actually have a chance to succeed.

Example:

Let's say, not to demean you in any way, you are currently 160 lbs. You have gone through all the weight calculators and have determined for your height and width you should weight 120lbs max. The difference is 40 lbs but that is also 25% of your current weight. That can be a lot for a start. A better strategy is to target 20 lbs.

Next, it is better to set up a time frame for reaching the target. This is not mandatory but is a good thing to do as it keeps the perspective of the whole effort within a visible boundary. However, it needs to be reasonable. If you can on average lose 1 lb a week then 20 lbs should take you about 20 weeks + 1 or 2 weeks. Give it 5 months. If you want to set up a tougher target you can do so but be advised that setting up high targets even though reachable may not always have a good long term effect. You may work really hard to meet your target but you will end up spending so much of your energy that the spirit and determination needed to maintain your prized body won't be there and you'll sooner or later dip into the regaining cycle.

Set your goals in a way so that you can comfortably meet it, comfortably does not mean without taking any effort, it simply means *not too much stress*. Having said it, if you feel that you have so much to lose that getting into such a leisurely pace may not do any good to you then think twice. One of the primary targets of any weight loss program should be:

Losing weight and keeping it lost

Being slow is not a problem, what is most important is maintaining the loss.

Maintain

If you are obese and have tried all kind of dieting, physical exercises and yet had little result, give it another try with me. Forget about the past. Just follow me...take it easy...enjoy the process...you'll lose weight and you'll be at your target one day.

The primary target of my program is simple

It is not only about losing weight. What is more important is to create a lifestyle that allows you to continue to lose weight, remain healthy and possibly happy. If you are not having any fun while you lose weight what good does it bring to you and your family and friends?

My motto:

Adjusting lifestyle = slow and steady changes without losing anything else but weight.

Don't be alarmed. The term *adjusting lifestyle* is used in a light way. It is not about changing your life. In most cases you still live your regular life with some necessary changes to accommodate your new effort. This could be modifying your sleeping pattern to your eating habits. We'll discuss those things in due time.

Chapter 4

Before we start

Knowledge is the way

It is important to have necessary knowledge about your approach. However, knowing can be quite confusing sometimes especially of a topic that have so much text floating around everywhere we look – starting from books to internet journals to user forums. Searching in the net with a keyword may ooze out too much information. Often it is not very helpful as a guiding source. It is also not easy to know about the authenticity of the information.

Anyway, the idea is to collect as much information as needed from authentic looking sources. Overdoing it may not do too much good as it can easily become exhausting, often confusing and possibly contradicting.

In this book I'll pass on whatever information you need to know to succeed in this relatively leisurely but effective approach. My request to you will be to ensure that you do not lose yourself in the jungle of information. Some are simply what people thinks, while some others are from experts who have certain interest in whatever they preach like a medicine, herbal stuff, an exercise instrument, a so called weight loss system etc. etc. There are plenty of those around now.

I have nothing else to sell beside this book. And this book contains everything that I have found through over fifteen years of personal attempts on this. The reason I bring this up is because I need your undivided attention. I need you not to veer away from it because suddenly you think you found a better procedure, a better remedy. Believe me when I say this – there's nothing called a better remedy. They are just made to look or feel like that. So, what is the summary of this section?

Knowledge is good but watch for nonsense.

Make up your mind and stick to it.

You may be wondering why I am hammering you with this basic stuff. You are smart and you know what is good for you. Point taken. If you weren't smart and health conscious you wouldn't be reading this book. The reason I am touching these points because often it is important to establish some very basic rules before going further. It helps with focus and determination, increasing the chances of success.

Socrates had taught '**Know thyself**'. Many people will explain that in many different ways. It is only couple of words but it touches the core of our identity. Because each one of us have different views and understandings of our identities and we do not necessarily always consider 'knowing thyself' to be *knowing* the same set of things. I, at this point, would want you to look at yourself from a very different perspective – the things that you'll need to succeed:

- *Patience*
- *Stubbornness*
- *Flexibility*
- *Tolerance*
- *Endurance*

I know, I know, these are all the good virtues that we all need to succeed in life. Fortunately, these good virtues are also the ones that will help you to succeed in your current quest, if you are taking it as a quest. If not then all you are going to get at the end is the *smile* with no loss of weight. That is not what we are trying to do here. I recommend you to do the following:

a. **Self Assessment**: *In a scale of 1 to 10 grade yourself in each of the virtues mentioned above [take as much time as you need]*

b. **Analysis**: *Pay special interest to any item that you feel you have a score less than 7. Create another list identifying why you scored yourself below 7 in those areas. Remember, you are not trying to lose some quick pounds. This is going to be your way of life. You can't continue in that path unless you have a very clear understanding of your limits and shortcomings. Your weight is not just a bunch of meat and fat, it is something that you have acquired either by overeating or simply by leading a way of life that did not work very well for you. There are people who could care less about their weight and the size of their waists; you definitely are* *not one of them. Please spend as much time as you need to examine the areas where you feel you are not up to par and create a detail list on your understanding of the underlying causes.*

c. **<u>Review</u>:** *Now, this is getting really interesting. Have at least two people score you separately on each of those categories. Compare the results with your own perception of you. You surely already figured out how that comparison can shape up to provide you a nice look at yourself*

     i.   *If the average of those two scores are within 10% of your own assessment then consider them matching. Good work!*

    ii.   *If the difference is larger than that then dig into it. Find out why your perception about yourself was different than the two scorers. How would that help? By simply giving you true insight into yourself. It'll allow you to know if you are as strong a person you think you are in the eyes of others. Are you seen to be flexible? Are you seen to be tolerant? All these virtues are needed to succeed.* **You'll be losing weight for days, months, years to come and will be keeping it away for the rest of your life, hopefully. That's the real goal.** *To achieve that goal you need to know if you have it in you to succeed. If not then you need to work on those virtues in parallel to your effort to lose weight. No short cuts there, not if you are thinking long term.*

Know your surroundings

It is a general statement nonetheless very important. But what does it really mean by 'knowing your surroundings'? I am bringing this up because this is something that will have a serious impact on your attempt to lose something unwanted, something that will change your life not only in your eyes but in the eyes of others – close or distant. Here are the things that I suggest you consider doing to evaluate your standing:

d. **Home**: How you live has a significant impact on your mentality and morality. It also in a way may affect your determination and tolerance.

e. **Family**: Take a good look at the close kin of yours whether they live with you or away from you. For obvious reasons they have a great impact on everything we do. They can lead us to great success. They can also push us to total failure. It is the reality of things that not all among us turn out to be same, even when there are equal opportunities. That`s how we humans are. Too many factors starting from genes, environment, upbringing, friend circle, political situation – I can keep going – can have an impact. But despite all that most of us come out as descent human being. If you cannot clearly label your surrounding as **descent or good** then perhaps you have something little more to work on then just weight. I don't mean that you still cannot succeed, but it simply would make things more challenging for you. If you are living among a group of people who could care less about looking lean and fit, it could in turn take away your motivation. Not saying it will but it definitely can. It has that potential. Perhaps you might try to convince some of them to work together with you in trying out this procedure.

f. **Friends**: Friends are probably the most important part during our adult life. Often they not only provide companion and support but also guide us in particular directions which may or may not be the best for us. Some people are strong enough to break out of negative influences but some cannot. This is why it is very important that you evaluate your friendship with all your close friends and determine who would be more or less helpful to you in your new quest. The more supportive they are the better – of course. Anybody who is dismissive of the idea it may be better to stay at a distance from that person for a little while, until you find your rhythm and get used to the routine. At that point your determination and mental strength would be at a level where it would be difficult to shift you from your target.

You must not compromise your happiness by any means just because you want to lose weight.

Once you have lost weight who are you going to hang on with? Your friends and family – of course. So, while you want to be careful and selective about whom you want to keep company with for a little while as you get settled in the program *it is also important to ensure that you do not mess up your relationship with anybody*.

Friends often need to be reminded that they are your friends in the first place and were expected to help you in making your life change for better. Any other way and the definition do not fit. You may even have to at times create a workable routine that would allow you to keep the friendship going while providing you with ample time to continue with your agenda. It may not be easy always, much tougher than saying for sure, but it must be done. And it must be done carefully, gently and in a well thought manner. Friends can be very touchy at times. You definitely don't want to hurt them. Do not get carried on. Keep your friends. You'll need them in every step of this journey. Sometimes you'll be tired, often disappointed, disheartened and even dejected. Sometimes you may even be at total loss of confidence, drowned in frustration and about to give up. I won't be with you, my words will, but that is not always very efficient when the feeling of frustration surpasses a threshold. It'll be your friends who can help you move through those pressing times.

Chapter 5

Phase 1

The beginning

Okay, we have covered a whole lot by now, but have not yet lost even an ounce of weight. I realize that. It was part of the plan. Remember what I had repeatedly said? **Losing weight is not just about losing weight.** It is much more than that. Even more if you want to do this while truly enjoying the process.

<u>I want to see you all smile while you are at it!</u>

I am not kidding. Happiness is what really should be guiding you. Not the other way around. There are many people out there who have tons of money but nothing to live for. Some of them even resort to ending their own lives. Shouldn't money take care of all that petty happiness related issues? Apparently not. That's why the first thing that I ask you to do, again and again, is to promise to yourself that no matter what you will not lose your happiness.

Good. Now let's step into phase 1 – taking care of the little nuisance called extra weight.

A few words about weight:

It is important to understand how our body works when it comes to weight. Knowing and Understanding the basics will help you all through your life.

The term **Metabolism** is so ominous now that it would be hard not to hear about it. Almost everybody are an expert when it comes to metabolism and if you pay a little attention you'll be surprised to find out how differing views people have about it. It takes no telling that many either do not have a clear understanding or are simply misguided. Believing in concepts like -

'I am overweight because my body has much less metabolism'

and/or

's/he is so thin even though s/he gorges on food because s/he has higher metabolism'

- are simply wrong. Not to say that s/he cannot have higher metabolism than you but that alone cannot be the cause of you being overweight and her/him being skinny, by no means. You need to look into other factors if you really are keen to find out the root cause, like food intake, lifestyle, activities, gender etc.

So, how is metabolism defined? It is a term used to express how much calorie – unit of energy - our body loses in a given time. I'll explain the concept behind this in details soon. When you read on a nutrition tag 'based on 2000 calorie diet' all that it says is that a normal person with normal activities would require 2000 calories to maintain their current weight. A part of that calorie need is caused by our metabolism.

To understand metabolism in details please refer to **Appendix A**. It may be a good idea to check it out first before continuing.

Usually daily metabolism is measured in terms of total calories that a normal adult person would consume in a day to maintain his weight, which is approximately 2000 calories. However, the required calorie differs heavily based on size, shape, activity and life style and also on gender. There are many online calculators to find out required calorie need. It is very important to find out the calorie need based on your average activities in a week. To find out your daily calorie need go to **Appendix B.**

Whatever number you get is not going to be fixed as you'll get more active and possibly more physically fit during the coming days as you continue into this effort. Do remember the following though

a) Once you start losing weight and become lighter your overall Basal metabolism (the calorie requirement to keep very basics of your body functions moving) may go down as its relationship with the body is with the total mass. You may already know brain is the organ that uses up most of the energy (17% or so). The rest goes to other organs and cells etc.

b) Just because you start looking leaner and possibly fitter doesn't mean your overall calorie requirement will go up. If you are not living a very physically active life style it is unlikely that your body would require drastically more calorie than before. The reason I mention this here is because from my observation I have noticed that once a person loses some weight s/he tend to increase her/his food intake believing that her/his body is now ready to burn the extra calories. This often is incorrect and people end up quickly gaining back.

Once you have a clear idea on your body's requirement of food on average per day (measured based on a weekly consumption pattern) now you can start doing some easy but quite interesting Math. I encourage you strongly to spend the time to do such calculations even though they are just that - calculations and may not be always very achievable. But let's not forget

Planning is important to succeed

no matter what we do.

The basic idea is ***3500 calories translates to 1 pound of mass in our body*** – overlooking all other criteria. So, as you can clearly realize that to control your weight either you'll have to simply *keep your food intake low* or *burn extra calories* by performing heavy workouts. The outcome will be same – you'll lose a pound or so. Of course, it is next to impossible to continue either one of them over long period of time for two reasons:

a) **Boredom:** Boredom may become a serious issue. Being intelligent animals we are very prone to boredom when performing repetitive activities. Hence it is important for us to mix and match and try to keep everything in a nice jolly mixture of interesting and hard work.

b) **Anti-starvation mechanism:** Our body is also itself a pretty strong and intelligent mechanism. Often there are things it does automatically that we cannot truly control. There is a very effective and interesting means our body has to fight food shortage which is called – *anti-starvation mechanism*. As part of this our bodies turn down Resting Metabolic Rate (RMR) and start to preserve resources for long term strategy – primarily fat – as it stores calories much more efficiently than Carbohydrates and Proteins. The outcome of this effect is that if we reduce food intake too drastically or even in a particular pattern we may kick our body to get into this mode. As a result the rate of loss of body mass reduces noticeably from the earlier stages. *Talk about trouble!* Even our own body works against us when it comes to losing weight. But don't be disheartened. With diligent approach and slow advances it is quite easy to beat the anti-starvation mechanism of the body. Patience and diligence are the virtues of the time.

Now, going back to the calculation, you can spend some time determining what type of target you want to set for yourself. However, I must warn setting up big targets is almost unachievable when it comes to body mass. It is my observation that after the initial phase (which we'll discuss soon) a good target would be to plan for ***1 pound a week loss***. Even that may become difficult to maintain over a period of time but it still makes a good doable target. Losing more is possible by increasing the amount of workouts on regular basis but it is not recommended.

<u>Don't be desperate, be determined</u>
<u>and methodical.</u>

Losing a pound a week equates to an average of 500 calories per day less than what our body needs to maintain current mass which is for adults roughly 2000 calories. There are three things you can do:

a) Reduce your food intake by 500 calories (this is not too much but may become difficult initially)

b) Perform physical activities to burn out the extra 500 calories. This I doubt can be done on a regular basis, true even for the most determined.

c) Reduce your food intake by 300 calories and burn out extra 200 calories by doing various exercises and activities, which we'll discuss in due time. *This is really the best plan.* However, there are many who may not be able to exercise owing to various reasons. For them the choice is obviously to reduce food intake.

Start easy:

One of the main problems with weight loss programs is that if it fails to show immediate and quick result, no matter how little, most people lose interest and faith in it. Almost everybody start with a lot of eagerness and spirit hoping to shed some quick pounds. The attitude is almost always like – *okay, now that I am eating only like half of what I used to eat before and also working out for a whole twenty minutes my extra weight should drop off like they are yesterdays garbage.*

Generally speaking, such quick initial weight loss is hard to achieve. Yes, sudden crash dieting may show some weight loss within one - two weeks but that is mainly caused by loss of water from the body and not much of fat. But the need for early visible loss is very, very important. I have actually seen people losing heart in just about two weeks after they failed to see any weight loss. I know it is not sustainable but yet I have resorted to a short term solution that can provide a kick start to the body and mind as an encouragement and allow a participant to settle down in the program by allowing some quick loss of mass. Please read on but very cautiously.

Atkin's diet

Robert Coleman Atkins, briefly known as Atkins, (October 17, 1930 – April 17, 2003) was an American physician and cardiologist. He had come up with a dietary solution of lowering carbohydrate consumption and emphasizing protein and fat as the primary sources of dietary calories. His approach is best known as 'Atkins Diet'. It is a popular but controversial way of eating.

[For details please refer to Appendix F]

Let's briefly analyze what this is all about.

At the core of Atkins diet is to reduce carbohydrate intake and resort to more meat (protein and fat) based diet to lose weight. There is some science behind this. Our body gets its energy initially from carbohydrate which we intake as part of our normal diet, then it moves to stored energy in the form of fat. Atkin suggested if we reduce carbohydrate intake then the body would have to get the required energy to run the body from burning fat. At the same time he suggested that because it took more energy to break down protein and fatty food a person burns more calories just by resorting to such diet.

While there are some truth to all his suggestions there are also contradictions and debates over protein and fat rich food intake over a longer period of time. It takes no telling that carbohydrate is what makes our food so full of variety. While fish and meat are good for our body too much of that may not be too good either as they put our body under higher stress to get digested.

Without getting too deep into that discussion or analysis I would lay out my suggestions:

- it is a common and clear observation that Atkin's meat based diet is very effective in reducing a few initial pounds quickly, as it causes our body to quickly lose some stored fat and water. The protein consumes more energy to be burned and may turn less into fat if eaten in reasonable quantity. But at the same time it is almost universally maintained that being on mainly protein diet for adult humans is not by any means a healthy approach as it tends to devoid the body of all the necessary vitamins and minerals. Also, not everybody can even tolerate such meat heavy diet, let alone those who abhore meat and resorts to vegeterian diet.

So, if you are not a vegan and is very keen on seeing some quick weight loss then adapt to Atkin's diet for about 3-4 weeks. I would suggest eating poultry, baking it instead of frying, especially avoid deep frying as it would contain a lot of fat from oil. Also, eat only reasonable portion ensuring that your calorie intake is less than what you need to keep your current weight. Depending on how you have laid down your plan on losing weight you must act accordingly. Once again, *planning is important.*

Are you a Vegan?

Now, if you are a vegan then you are already doing something right. Just ensure that you control your carbohydrate intake. By managing your rice, bread or other grain food intake you can reduce a lot of calorie consumption. The idea is again to have less calorie than you normaly need to maintain your body. You may not get the doubtful advantage of the jump start with Atkins diet but you can easily compensate for that by doing slightly more workout (are you starting to lose your smile now that I have mentioned the dreaded workout?). Don't be afraid, I do not propose that you start doing serious work out at this point. If you are already into exercise then I won't ask you to stop or slow down. Though I personally do not recommend too much of physical exercise as I have seen from my experience practically everybody at some point gets tired of extensive workout and become suddenly laid back, which does not help by any means. Anyway, we'll discuss that in details a little later.

The initial 3-4 weeks - Summary

- If you are comfortable with it do the meat routine for two to three weeks. It shows some quick pound loss and usually works as a psychological booster. If you don't want to do it so be it. Go to next topic.

- Find out your required calorie intake. Eat 400-500 calorie less each day. We'll discuss soon on how to reduce that much calorie intake without difficulties in coping with it.

- If you are already doing exercise continue to do so. However, keep it within reasonable limit. Don't go overboard. If you are not doing any exercise then you may plan to start, slowly. We'll cover soon what kind of exercise is going to be better for you in this initial period.

Calorie picking:

This topic by itself can be a complete book. But it is not my intention to give it more importance than it should receive for our purpose. No, I do not mean to sound as if I don't think it is a very significant part of our plan. However, it is my observation that sometimes people loses focus and gets too taken by all the food choices. Too much of anything is usually not good. While there are many experts with different opinions a general guideline about food is to balance it in the following manner:

Protein

Carbohydrate

Fat

Saturated fat

Mono- saturated fat

Fiber: Soluble/non soluble etc.

Some of your daily food intake could be as below:

[Based on what is your daily routine you may be big on breakfast and light on supper or vice versa. I am a night owl. I rarely eat breakfast, have a light lunch and eat a big supper with four – five hours to burn it before I hit the bed. Many are just opposite. They are up early; eat a nice breakfast, a reasonable lunch and a light supper. Whatever works for you, it is you who'll have to decide. The below is an example only.]

Breakfast: [500 calories] 2 loafs of bread with jam/ jelly/ egg/spreads, a cup of milk or juice, a cup of coffee or tea with one milk and one sugar.

The choices would also depend on your physical condition. If you have cholesterol then it is probably a good idea to keep the eggs not more than 2-3/week. With diabetes too much sugary food may not be in your best interest. Also not all juices are suitable in every condition. An example would be grapefruit juices which may not be a good choice during pregnancy. You'll need to look at all the choices with proper knowledge and determine what and how you want to eat keeping it within the rough calorie limit.

Lunch: [500 Calories]

If you had a moderate breakfast then a light lunch is the best. By light I mean really light. A sandwich would work fine. Whole grain would provide some good fiber. Use fat free or low fat meat, vegetable inside the sandwich. Some sort of spread may work well too. I have successfully used Nutella for many years. Two teaspoon of Nutella or something of that nature can be very delicious and not too heavy in calories. Please be aware that Nutella or products like that should be eaten in a very small amount as they may contain high amount of fat and sugar. Also, I do not suggest any particular product. I mentioned Nutella as it worked very well for me.

The best way to handle this is to look around to see what would work well for you. Deli sandwich could be a good choice too. Smoked meat usually is lean and contains fewer calories while is very delicious.

Fruits may also work well though it should be noted that too much fruits may not be a very healthy practice either. I would suggest eating something with grains and then eat a piece of fruit about two – three hours later. This would keep you full until dinner time.

Dinner: [800]

While the dinner/supper time would depend on your personal habit if you are in a situation where you are trying to lose weight it probably is a good idea to eat early. Eating a full meal as oppose to smaller meals is usually a good idea as this will ensure couple of things

- You won't be consuming some unnecessary calories in the form of snacks, often high calorie ones like potato chips.

- Going to bed little early would mean that instead of being hungry you'll be sleeping and there won't be any need for eating. However, one thing to remember here is that you should keep at least two-three hours after a meal before going to bed. That way the food has enough time to get digested.

As for what to eat, try to stay within the allocated calorie limit. 800 calories may not be very much but it is not very little either.

- Alternate between carbohydrate/protein based main dish along with some vegetables, preferably not fried. Cook with water to keep the oil calorie out of it. However, it is also important to make the food as tasty as possible while trying to keep the calories low. If you do not enjoy the food, it is unlikely that you would continue to eat it.

- Cucumber, lettuce and tomatoes are great low calorie but filling stuff to eat as salad before the meal. They would usually take out some of the appetite. It is advisable to make the salad as delicious as possible to keep it interesting over long period of time.

- Another very useful technique is to eat slowly relishing whatever you are eating. There is a science behind this as well.

  - It takes our brain about 20 minute to get the signal that we are full. Often we eat too quickly, not allowing this subtle procedure to take place in time. As a result we end up eating way more than what would normally be enough.

- It is also preferable to come up with various menus and vary the food. Baking or grilled are definitely great way to keep the fat out.
- Do remember, we also need some fat from our diet. So, there's no need to be too crazy about keeping fat away. Just a reasonably conscious way works best.
- Baked or smoked fish is also great idea.
- Grilled vegetables, kebabs etc are good choices too.

For a detail list with calories refer to **Appendix D**

Light exercise:

Now let's get into more interesting areas of this journey. Before getting into any details I would like to stress on the fact that the main driving force to losing weight is to keep the food intake low or in another words – **counting calories**. Exercise is complementary, not the primary means. It has been observed in studies that the fastest and most effective way of losing weight is to do moderate dieting with moderate workout. Moderate is important in the beginning because very hard workout may actually become a boomerang. It can in turn make you hungrier and force you to eat more. As a result you may lose more energy but you'll take in much more than you lost. It is a very common mistake many beginner weight watchers do.

Burning calories are much harder than eating calories. It takes almost an hour of jogging to burn five hundred calories. A piece of cake contains about that many calories. It takes one minute to eat one.

Nevertheless, workout is very important because it not only burn calories, it also give your body the much needed boost. This can work toward increasing metabolism, making us feel better, providing us with the much needed feel good hormones. But it is also important to know what type of work out would work well in the beginning. In the following section I'll be discussing about some of the preferred workouts that I suggest for the beginners.

Before getting into more details I would like to emphasize on the fact that there are varieties of workout. Each can be targeted for different outcomes. While all of them are good for the body this way or that way it is important to understand your own needs and make a plan accordingly. At this point your sole goal is to lose weight. Hence we need to plan something that will help with losing weight faster and steadily.

It has been determined after many experiments that the best way to burn fat is to do workouts that do not need very high level of energy too quickly. Because what that does is burn the glucose in our body as oppose to fat to meet the immediate need. It is a good idea to start thinking of your body as an intelligent factory that already has a lot of the things going quite right. And it always works for the benefit of your body. It stores fat to save you from future starvation; it also tries to hang on to it as long as it can. It acts that way for your own good. Unfortunately, when you are trying to lose weight such mechanism may actually in a way work against you.

Anyway, at this early stage it is better that **you either jog or walk fast** for at least 30 to 60 minutes. You can do it outside or indoor on a treadmill. Often a treadmill works better as it allows seeing how fast you are going and the amount of energy burnt. You can also modify the settings to change the workout conditions. At the same time, if doing indoor, you can watch TV or even have conversations with your family members. The idea is to do it for longer time without getting bored and keeping your heart rate around 120 beats per minute. That is the optimal condition for most % fat burned. And fortunately, it doesn't take too much to reach that level.

Some of the other exercises that you can do are: **biking, elliptical**.

From my personal experience I feel elliptical can be a very good equipment to provide a kick start as you are trying to get used to the process. This equipment works using your own weight. As a result the knees do not get much pressure. That is a very positive thing. It instantly takes away the impression of hard work and pain of workout and provides an easy looking, fun type thing to do. Every gym has several of these machines. Do keep in mind that the displays on these machines like many others are set to show slightly increased calorie burned values.

Always deduct 15% of what the machines shows you have burnt.

Believe it or not the manufacturers intentionally do that because they have data to show people like to see that and it increases their sales. Unfortunately seeing higher than real numbers would not help you in any way. Instead it would give you a wrong impression and you may end up eating more thinking you have burnt more. Just to be on the safe side, make a habit of doing this.

To get a good understanding of various types of exercises versus calories burnt please refer to **Appendix E.**

Chapter 6

Phase 1 - Start

Start of week 1:

Like anything else an official start date and time may not be a very bad idea for starting a self help weight loss program. Why? It gives seriousness to the whole process and prepares the mind and body for something worthy. While it is greatly possible that you might have to revisit the same pattern of weight loss (after failing few times) it still is a good idea to have a start date every time you restart.

I like start of the working week to coincide with starting things that are kind of important. It helps keeping track of the progress better having weekdays and weekend to separate things. Often working hard during the weekdays and letting slightly lose in the weekends may work for some individuals. But we'll talk about that later in details.

Monday is the start day

Week 1 routines

We have practically covered everything that you'll be doing. Let's cover them quickly once more:

1) **Dieting** – Reduce food intake. Your target is to eat five hundred calories less than your normal calorie intake. Initially this is a great target. Ensure that you go through the food calories and create your own nice list of food (including fruits) that you want to eat and stay within the limit. In addition don't forget to keep an eye on the nutritional values.

2) **Workout** – Start doing some simple workouts like walking for half an hour. Do not push yourself so early. Just let your body slowly get used to all this.

3) **Chill** – Take it easy. Remember you are not in it for a few weeks. Get settled for long term commitment. That is why it is so important to take things easy and to enjoy.

4) **Keep yourself busy -** The busier you remain the better you'll do. Work often makes people forget about their hunger. That is a good thing.

End of week 1

It is very important to take a break from the routine of weight loss program. Whether you are taking a softer approach or harder approach would matter little when you come to making sure that your body and mind both get rested sufficiently so that you can start all over again when the new week starts.

These are some of the things that each individual should be able to create based on his or her ability and mind set. A general direction is to have a mild freedom and not binge on food or drink. The basic principle of building a modified life style still stands. Hence it is definitely not advisable to engage into things that can easily cause some headache when the time comes to get back into the routine on Monday morning. So the motto should be

Enjoy without breaking

The idea is simple as you must have already figured it out. Your body needs some kind of relief from the tight and possibly difficult schedule where you are rationing everything from food to drink to activities. Not something that we really appreciate. However, the break shouldn't be too long, definitely not for the whole of the weekend. The basic calculation would still stand: every 3500 calories equates to 1 pound of mass. You burn the calories you lose a pound and vice versa. The reality of the matter is burning 3500 calories is way harder than eating 3500 extra calories (at the top of what our body requires). A large piece of cheese cake is easily 500 calories. If you are used to drinking wine or liquor there are considerable amount of calories in them. Any type of non diet carbonated drink has considerable amount of calories from sugar. If you are not watching out you may go overboard very easily.

If you like to eat in restaurants, especially buffet, you may easily go way past your food requirement and gorge way beyond your need. A Chinese buffet may add 5000 calories in one meal if you truly enjoy the greasy, sugary delicious foods. I do, even now. There was a time when I used to go for the Chinese and Indian buffet at least once a week. There's little need to say how it turned out for me. I packed up more than 10 pounds some months. I loved the food, even after knowing all the bad things they contained. I still do, but instead of going once a week now I go once every four months. However, when I do go I gorge in a way as if there is no tomorrow. Fortunately my stomach have shrunk quite a bit and a serious consciousness about managing my weight roams my mind all the time, hence even at my worst I am nowhere near breaking my old records.

Math all the time

Whatever you eat, whatever you plan to eat and drink, always do calculation at the back of your mind. Ensure you take the time to remember roughly the calorie content of most food you eat, try to come up with the rough number of total calories that you are going to eat even before you consume. We tend to under do such calculation as in our subconscious mind we are simply waiting to indulge us. Hence, **spend some time to determine exactly what % calorie you under calculate**. My guess is this number should be within 25-50% range. Which means when something has a real calorie content of 300, we might erroneously believe that it has 150 to 200 calories. Compensate for such low balling after each calculation.

Meals

When it comes to main meals you'll hear lots of different ideas catering to all kind of views and even medical findings. Some would suggest you have a big meal and nothing thereafter, others would suggest you eat in small quantities but many times a day. While there cannot be any one way to do this it is important to realize that regardless of how you eat the governing force should still be the calorie count. One really big meal or three small meals would not make much difference if at the end both the calorie content matches, generally speaking.

Let's be frank, food is not always about hunger. Often food is more mental than physical. To elaborate we don't eat just to respond to our hunger but also because we like the taste, the aroma and above all the complete experience of eating. How we consume our daily calories would not matter much as long as we remain within our limits and enjoy the experience. It is important to relish the food we eat. The motto should be – **quality not quantity.**

Again, the choice of few big meals or small frequent meals is really a personal one. I prefer eating one big meal each day, perhaps two in the weekends. For me it works pretty well as with my stomach full my urge for eating goes away for several hours allowing me to concentrate on other things. Drinking some water at regular intervals keep the system hydrated. However, **too much water is not recommended.** Especially do not use water to fill up your empty stomach hoping that would help you curb your hunger. It usually doesn't work and may even cause bodily discomfort.

Very light snacks may be eaten in between meals. However, what is light? Most snacks are heavy on calories, especially the appetizing ones. You must use your judgment. A snack should not go too much over 100 calories, which may not provide much nutrition depending on type of food. In terms of potato chips it would be about 10 chips. It is never easy to eat only ten of those delicious treats. Use control. Sometimes try cucumber, tomatoes, lettuce, bell paper etc. with dip. If you are not used to eating salad it would take a little practice but eventually you'll start to like them. Use a good dressing or dip to make them more appetizing. Of course that would add some more calories but still much better than packaged high calorie, high fat choices. Try fat free dressing or dip if you can tolerate it.

Before moving out of this topic lets visit the cons for each proposed eating method.

- People eating one or two big meals may eat too much at once and feel uncomfortable later. It is important to determine how much is enough.
- People eating several small meals often tend to miscalculate their food intake and end up eating more calories. As discussed before many snacks are very high on calories but little on quantity. This may result in feeling of hunger even though enough calories have been consumed.

Snacks:

We'll talk about meals more in details later. For now let's get the case of snacks out of our way.

Snacks may be considered differently in different parts of the world, or even in different families. In some countries a snack can be as big as a meal. However, standard definition is probably smaller quantity and as a result less food energy. I would define it to be anywhere less than 200 calories. Any more than that and it should not be considered as a snack. It may help to remember that a snack really is to carry you until the next big meal.

There are plenty of options when it comes to snacks. You just need to make sure that you are reading the calorie contents and the nutrition values. One thing do bear in mind that

Low calorie snacks sucks! (Generally speaking)

However, with time and effort it is possible to get used to the intolerable. We must be adamant, persisting. A little imaginative or being creative definitely helps. My suggestion is slightly different than you may be thinking...

Eat the delicious, high calorie snacks sometimes, just eat very little.

Enjoy the taste of it, chew it slowly, and relish it as long as you can – just don't eat too much. A little food when eaten properly can go a long way. Eating too much too quick provides less pleasure and contentment. Eating is an art. Once you get it deep inside your mind, you won't have to worry about eating too much. There simply won't be a need. The joy and pleasure that you'll be able to capture from one bite could take another person a whole serving.

For some ideas look into **Appendix C.**

How to lose appetite:

What to do to stop thinking about food?

Tough question. Primarily because each one of us are different to some extent. Not the same things interest us or entertain us. But, still we can come up with some general suggestions which may work as a starting point. I might even dare to say that there are some techniques that can be considered universal. Let's dig into it a little.

- **Get busy:** Getting engaged in something that you really enjoy doing is probably one of the best ways to keep thought of foods at the back of your mind. This, unfortunately, can also be computer games, video games etc. I say _unfortunately_ because such games can also become very addictive and may hurt in other areas but they do work to hold complete attention. Just make sure you are not eating as you play.

- **Work:** No matter whatever we do for a living any type of work can be very engaging. If you are an office worker like me take lunch from home and make sure it is just enough to keep you going until you return home. Also, no matter how bad you look try to avoid going out to eat lunch from work with your colleagues. I admit sometimes it does get very tempting. But fighting temptation is the best way to win this war. Just tell yourself you must do with whatever little food you have brought from home. First few days this may be painful but over time this will work very well. Remember, at the end of the day you'll have saved enough calories for a nice dinner/supper.

- **Keep food away** – This is another very good technique. You must remember the proverb 'out of sight out of mind'. It does work with food. Keep them out of your sight, if necessary hide them, put them in a place where you can't reach easily. Of course you won't be able to do it with all type of foods. But this works great with snacks like chips, cookies and other stuff that fall in that category. Usually these are the food that we eat without realizing how much we have eaten. If you can't stay away from them, keep them away from you – out of sight of you.

- **Buy enough only** – Often we get good sales and end up buying way more than we can consume quickly. As a result we end up eating more thinking this is the only way to utilize the extra purchase. Cheap stuff is good but don't buy unless you really need them.

- **Resist yourself** – Perhaps this is the most important thing. No matter how little food we buy and how well we hide them we would still get tempted at some point and would look for food. If you must give in to temptation try to keep it low. If you must eat potato chips eat 5 or at most 10. Resisting isn't as difficult as it sounds. You must not give in too easily. Fight back!

How to get into the Mode?

What can be done to ensure successful transition to weight loss mode?

Perhaps the most important part of this complete effort is to getting into appropriate state of mind or briefly **mode**. Losing weight, I am sure anybody who have been trying it already knows, is a true question of *self motivation*.

No matter what others say and how they say it, unless one succeeds in creating an overwhelming urge to lose weight, it is never going to happen.

But the question is how to *feel that urge*? Or a more appropriate question could be how to *enhance that urge*?

Different things work for different people especially when it comes to motivation. Still it may be possible to suggest some general approach which individually or collectively may work.

(a) **Look yourself at the mirror**: Often this could create the strongest of all motivation. If you don't like what you see then you are halfway down there. However, if it is a hesitating 'no' or 'what *the heck'/'who cares'* then we have a problem. None of those works well to generate motivation.

(b) **Do you feel good about yourself**: Do you feel comfortable with the way you carry your physical appearance? Again if the answer is a quick *'No'* then it would definitely get easy to start. Otherwise, need to resort to other techniques to bring in the elusive motivation.

(c) **Do you like the way others treat you:** based on your physical appearance, do you feel you are being treated with respect? This one can sometimes be a tough sale. Often people may not be in a perfect shape but due to their pleasant personality or for other reasons may look perfectly fine to others. That can be in a way bad as a motivating factor as it really does just the opposite. The only thing I can suggest is if you have decided for whatever reasons to lose some weight don't let such things stand on your way. Remember if they like you today there is no reason to believe that they won't tomorrow. If it turns out that people do have strong opinion about your appearance then it is a better idea to use that to motivate you instead of using the lame logic '*I don't care what they say*'. In most cases what others say do have some ground.

(d) Do you feel you are a strong enough person to do it? When nothing works this might. Here you are ignoring all other facts and simply trying to push your own ego to help you get sufficiently motivated to start the program. Whether it alone is strong enough to carry you all the way remains to be seen but this could definitely provide you the much needed first push.

How to carry on?

Let's not fool ourselves. Losing weight, quit smoking, stop taking drugs are all extremely difficult things to do. While one might think that losing weight has nothing to do with addiction of tobacco or drugs the truth is eating can be the worst of all addictions because it is one thing that seems perfectly safe. Think about all the foods that you consider your favorites. Can you smell the aroma, taste the deliciousness and see the appetizing image of it in your mind? The truth is just thinking of good food can be like sex, pleasing and satisfying in just about every way. Now consider this, how many of us can control our urge to eat up to our throat when we have access to all the food that we truly love? Only a few can. That's how most human are – call it a weakness or specialty.

So the question that we must tackle at this point is:

How can we win over this constant urge about eating?

This is a tough question. Again different things may work for different people. But generally there are a few things that may help. I have discussed a few little ago. Let's take another look at it.

(a) **Convince yourself that** somehow you just need to continue this painful process for 2 to 3 weeks. After that it would become normal and there will be no pain or less pain.

(b) **Find something to keep yourself busy**. This can be computer games, video games, creative work, social work, voluntary work, professional work etc.

(c) **Reading often is a great way** to keep one's mind away from the temptation of food. Or movies. Videos. Find out what works for you. There got to be something or several things.

(d) Keep the food hidden and scarce. It is a fact of life that most human being are impulsive eaters. If we see a delicious food lying there to be eaten most of us would probably take a bite – some big some small. Best is to totally keep it out of sight.

(e) Count days as you continue to abstinent (or try to do so). Remember 2 to 3 weeks are the painful period. After that things will get better. That is really your strongest motivator. Why? Because it is easily achievable.

Okay, so let's leave it there. Some of the stuff were repetitive but guess what, _repeating in this business is probably the best way to achieve any result_.

Anyway, let's assume you are doing all the right things. You are fighting with your craving for food; you are keeping yourself busy and engaged; you are not making any impulsive food purchases. Great! See you in a week or two.

Just in case things don't go very well in the first week, don't give up. Just start over and take an additional week. When you feel you are willingly (or unwillingly) sticking to the program then you may consider yourself ready for the next stage of this journey.

Chapter 7

Phase 2

Add little exercise to the mix

So, you have done the first thing – successfully reduced your food intake to some extent. I do not expect you to starve, that won't be good. Hopefully you are still eating, just a smaller portions. I am also hoping it has been about **three weeks** since you started this program, marching on all by yourself and may be with a little help from me in the form of motivation. It is important to let that dieting thing to sink in for a few days before starting on something new. By new, at this point I am inevitably referring to workouts.

Okay, I am assuming you are not too much into workouts, at least not recently. Usually people who regularly exercise are less likely to have serious weight issues, generally speaking. Personally I have noticed when I stop doing regular workouts I start to slide – on all level.

Food intake goes up; coupled with relatively inactive life style I start to become chubby. What is the message here? It is very important to add some form and amount of exercise with the dieting to truly achieve your goal – **be fit and healthy and of course shed some extra pounds in the process.**

If you have a past of sportsmanship or being part of fitness programs or things of that nature you probably already know all sorts of things about exercise and related stuff. Just in case you are not one of the sportsperson here is what I can advice you. If you follow them as is or with some modifications you should expect to see some result. Okay, let's get a little deeper into this.

What kind of exercise?

Nowadays exercise is a very vast thing – with so many options, facilities and expertise around and easily available. However, having too much resources and options around are not always a good thing. To a novice or uninformed or improperly informed it can easily become a daunting task to figure out what would be best or suitable for his/her needs. Yes, you can go to a gym and pay to become a member. Some gyms have instructors who can definitely help you to some extent though often they may not fully understand your particular need. You may also include yourself in various types of other related activities like dancing, martial art, yoga etc. Do whatever works for you.

However, I suggest if this is your first time trying out this particular procedure to lose weight do not join anything where you'll be too tired or exasperated. In the initial stages of weight loss effort it is simply not a good idea. Remember, we want to take it easy. By easy I mean not stressing yourself up too much too quickly. We'll get to the *stress yourself* part when the time comes. So, what are my suggestions? Here they go. Please do consider them regardless of your level of previous knowledge and experience with workouts:

(a) **Start with light exercise**. Here are some of them:

   a. **Slow jogging** – start with 10 minutes. Increase slowly over time as you continue to feel comfortable. But at no point allow your muscles to overwork. Remember, painful muscle would mean staying away from workout. That would simply mean losing the tempo, which can in turn become a horrendous mistake. Losing tempo could sometimes mean not being able to get back to it for months.

b. **Biking** – outdoor or stationary. Again, take it easy. Don't put too much strain on your body right away. Do it until you start to feel uncomfortable.

c. **Elliptical** – Do it in easy settings. This instrument is great for people who may have knee problems. All gyms now have it. Purchasing a good one could become expensive. However, a used one would work just fine. It has no electrical component beside display and is really easy on the joints.

d. **Walking** – while walking is a good thing for our body it is barely an exercise if not done in a considerably good pace. This can be done outdoor or on a treadmill. Do it for about 40 minutes. If necessary take small breaks.

e. **Swimming** – very good workout. Do it for at least 40 minutes, in little more than a leisurely pace.

(b) I suggest you *do not do* the following right away

a. **Do solely yoga**. It is great exercise but should be done in conjunction with one of the workouts I have mentioned before.

b. **Martial art** or similar stuff. Not just yet. In most cases such training could become too strenuous.

c. **Use heavy instruments** like weights or similar. Not at this point. All that would come but later.

How much?

Of course you are the best judge of your own body and would know your limits. But consider the following suggestions to determine the length of time and frequency of exercise:

(a) Do it three to five days a week. Take a break after two three days if you must. It is okay to do as many days as you feel like doing.

Remember we are not doing anything stressful. Muscle building exercises cannot be done on consecutive days. However, simple running, biking, swimming, walking type exercises can be done regularly as long as you are comfortable with it.

(b) **Do it for half an hour to one hour**. Start slowly. Perhaps with half an hour of walk. When you are comfortable and start to get the heck of it increase your duration and type, going for slightly more strenuous ones (but nothing to hurt yourself).

(c) **Do several type of exercise**, each at least for five minutes. If you are jogging add a few freehand workouts.

(d) **Do not do for too long at a time**. Not until much, much later. One hour is a good limit. Stay within that or close to that. Less is fine. More may not be good. Remember the more work out you do the hungrier you'll feel. That's not what your goal is. We want to jump start your body to get to a higher metabolism, not to get so hungry that you end up eating more (or spend all your energy in resisting the temptation).

When?

The actual time of the day for working out can be important too. While some people feels comfortable in the morning others may be more inclined to do so in the evening. However, lining it up with rest of your activities all through the day will actually bring in most benefit. What do I mean?

1. It is a **fact of life** that each one of us is more active at certain time of the day. Some are early risers and ready to shoot out for a jog, while some others can barely open their eyes before it is much later in the morning. They could actually be very active in the evening. It is definitely a good idea, if time permits, to work out when your body is most active.

2. If you **simply can't find time** to work out when you really feel like doing it choose the next best time. Possibly in the evening. If you are a working person and work during day time then the best time for you to exercise is in the evening. Not to

deny the fact that you will probably be pretty tired at that time. Take a short break. Don't eat anything heavy. Best is not to lie down. Don't allow your body to relax too much. After half an hour get to it (workout). You should be fine.

3. Exercising **too late at night** may not be a good idea as it can ruin your sleep, something that is not desirable at all. Getting good rest is at the core of everything you are doing.

4. Exercising **too early in the morning** may not be very good either. Especially not heavy workouts. Being tired in the morning may affect rest of your day. You may even feel hungry and lethargic.

What if I don't want to?

1. I don't suggest you push yourself to the point where the whole thing starts to feel like a *pressure*. That would not serve the purpose.

2. It is not necessary to exercise at all if you live an active life. What is an active life? You know what is a couch potato is. Try to find out your distance from that. The further you are the better. Just

pacing inside your house can give you enough workouts to boost your metabolism. Of course it is not as good as doing some slightly more strenuous exercise but it is definitely not bad.

3. If for whatever reason you feel neither exercise nor being active is your thing then do the inevitable. Focus on dieting only. Though I do not feel that alone can give you something that you can keep for long time but what else can you do? Dieting would still get the work done, if you can stick to it. You just have to do it in a much stricter fashion.

4. You may even join a gym and try doing some group workout. They are usually good to create some initial encouragement. If you can team up with your close friends or relatives that would definitely work in your favor.

Continue this for another three-four weeks.

For more information on different type of exercises and related calorie burning table check out **Appendix E**

Chapter 8

Phase 3

After three weeks (or so)

Okay, so you have successfully been in the program for three weeks now. Even if you had missed a few days here and there still as long as you feel you have been taking the effort and really enthusiastic about this whole experience then consider yourself *'in the right path'* and move on with the program.

Get into a rhythm: Let's check what you have achieved.

It is important to identify what you have succeeded in doing and what you felt didn't work as well as you had expected. My suggestion would be to actually make a written list.

The things that worked: *Your list.*

The things that did not work: *Your list.*

Obviously things that worked are good things to know. Because they are really your keys to success. Those are your strong sides. You know your strength and if necessary you can actually boost your effort in those areas to mitigate any risk caused by the areas where you are not as strong.

Of course, the areas where you failed provides you just as important information about yourself. You know where you need to work on. Often it may seem like difficult tasks to get it going but you'll be surprised once you made up your mind how you may actually win over your weaknesses. Let's consider a simple example. Many coffee and tea lovers are used to drink their beverages with lots of suger and milk. As part of their dieting program if they can learn to drink black, they can essentially save 50 – 100 calories per cup. If somebody is drinking 4-5 cups a day (say Tim Horton's double-double) the total saving almost equals to a meal. If you are a coffee or tea lover that can be one of the areas you want to work on.

Generally speaking, after three weeks it is time for

you to revisit all the effort you have taken and to see if it provided you with the outcome that you had expected to see when you started the program. Some of the areas that you need to evaluate your gains or losses are the following:

1. Have you actually lost any weight?
2. If you have how much?
3. Is the weight loss more/less/same as what you had planned for?
4. How do you feel overall going through this?
5. Do you feel this is something you can continue to do for say one year or until you have lost the weight that you have planned for?
6. How is your temperament? Are you too snappy? Peevish? Impatient?
7. How do you feel about your changed food habit?
8. How strong you feel your determination is at this point to continue?
9. How is your level of confidence?

Ask whatever question you want to ask yourself. The questions mentioned above were just some that I suggested. You should come up with appropriate set of questions so that you can figure out how your overall effort is going and whether it needs any adjustment.

Now the most important things to consider. Say, you just found out that things weren't going as you thought it would.

You are miserable.

You are in pain.

You are annoying, hungry and a total wreck.

All of those are possible. They can happen all together or partially. None of them can be ignored. I have personally seen several people who have really tried to continue, as long as they could, and then gave up. They weren't following my system – but they had the willingness to lose weight nonetheless.

Now, let's be honest. I don't want to be one of those coach who keep screaming *we must win*, *we must win* when nothing is working out. There are many areas in life where winning takes more than just will power and self determination. Circumstances may end up playing a much bigger role than we want it to be. Whatever it is, there are also some battles where the odds of succeeding is higher. Losing weight in my opinion falls in that second category. It is possible to do it. It has been done. It can be done. External influence may play a role but it can easily be defeated. That is one of the main reason why I would continue to push you to move forward and not to give up – no matter what.

Whatever happens do not give up. Giving up is easy, in anything. That exactly what most people does. They try a little bit and comes up with some rationale to simply give up. Don't be like them. Convince yourself that you are *more capable than others*. Show your strength. Prove yourself to you. Just thinking that you are stronger than others is usually a good way to boost your moral.

Let's consider another scenario. Say, you are generally okay with the program but not sure if it is being benefitial to you. In that case you may want to do some adjustment. If you have not lost reasonable amount of weight then obviously some tweaking is necessary to boost your effort.

Now, let's think about another scenario where you have done so well that you have not only reached your target but actually done so by enjoying the process. Great!

You are truly into it. Still there may be some need for adjustment.

I am assuming that you have sort of paid attention to whatever I have been saying and resorted to Atkin's diet for the initial few weeks. As I have explained this short Atkins diet would almost certainly provide a jump start to your weight loss effort. How much you lose would definitely depend on how desperate you are. My suggestion would be to take it easy. Nothing is good when you overdo it. If you have lost more than five pounds that is not unusual but be advised this rate will not persist week after week. Actually, with Atkin's diet weight loss would almost stop after several weeks. For the science behind it read the **appendix F**. Anyway, I guess you are starting to sense what I am about to say. <u>Do not continue on Atkin's diet for too long</u>. It is not considered to be a healthy dietary system by most dieticians and health care professionals. However, there are people on both ends when this particular dietary system comes. I have decided to favor the mixed dietary practices focusing primarily on vegetables, fruits and essential portions of meat and grains. I do not think getting used to abnormal food practice benefits at the long run.

So, if you have been three − four weeks or so on Atkins diet this is about time you snap out of it and start to get back to your regular diet − not quantity wise but quality wise. Best is to slowly merge the two. Reducing carbohydrate in the diet and inserting some meat is good.

You can do all kind of research at this point: talk to others, discuss with health specialists etc. There's nothing wrong with it. However, by now you know one thing for sure − it's you who have the power to make it work.

It is not a complex thing. It is not even very hard thing.

The only reason it has become a billion dollar business is because we don't show enough strength to take the proven but relatively long path and always look for shortcuts, miracles, easy looking solutions. Most of the time all the money that people spend on fancy workout programs are really more feel good type and often the little result they produce are easily lost as soon as there is an interruption, even a short one. I have seen too many people ending in complete failure.

Do the simplest of things:

1. Go slow and steady. You already know the

formula for weight loss: 3500 calories = 1 pound.

2. Count your calories.
3. Eat healthy but allow some freedom regularly
4. Don't stress yourself up too much
5. Don't allow long lapses

If it helps you should create a chart of what and how much you want to eat the whole week using calorie content and nutritional values of food of choice, planned work out amount and possible calorie burnt as a general guidance.

A common advice is to *relax every now and then to some extent. Eat the fatty icecream you have been craving for lately.* Or *the two donuts that you really wanted to have.* What bad is going to happen? Not much if you can keep in mind that sometime during that week you'll have to let go something else. Make it a **business of priorities**. It's really you vs you. You can make it work. Just don't do one thing – **never let go**.

As you slowly change your diet and life style to keep you content and energized while you continue to lose weight, albeit slowly, stop counting days. **Count only**

weeks.

If you want to check your achievements <u>do it once in a week.</u> If you are mentally strong and things seem to work then hopefully you'll continue to lose half a pound to one pound every week. **There is no need or benefit to try to do too much.** If you do very hard excercise and serious dieting then there is a possibility that you may be able to lose two three pounds regularly each week but I strongly advice against it. It is better to take it relatively easy and continue to *enjoy* your normal life. Of course the definition of *normal* must have changed somewhat by now but you get the idea. Being as close as possible to your normal life before you got into all this.

I am hoping that you are doing everything right and losing weight. I am also assuming at some point you will close on to your target. Whether that target is twenty pounds, fifty pounds, hundred pounds – doesn't matter. At some point you'll get there if you continue to live your new lifestyle. Don't spend too much money for weight loss. Don't overdo anything. Eat enough, drink enough (I don't drink any liquor and suggest against it but if you do drink don't forget liquor does have calories.) A bear probably have 70 to 120 caloties. Try to avoid it if you possibly can. If not drink little. The good things about it underweighs the bad things by heavy margin. Anyway, in the next chapter we'll talk about life after success. If, just in case, you fail at this point do not get disheartened. Take a short break and jump back in. Remember, it's your body. You have full control over it, generally speaking, and you can do it if you really are determined.

Chapter 9

What Can Go Wrong

Is there anything that cannot go wrong?

Like all good things during your attempt to lose weight one thing will happen amply – everything will tend to go wrong. From your mood to food, from feeling good to terrible, from 'everything going great' to 'what a crap' – trust me all of those are going to happen. Some days you would feel like going to the gym first thing in the morning, while some other days, most days, you wouldn't even want to think about moving your body in an unfavorable way. It happens not only to the starters, it actually happens to the experts more often than anybody else. Now of course 'experts' is used here slightly jocular way. There cannot be any expert weight losers. If you become an expert doing it then you should have been there already. However, there can definitely be expert weight watchers. Once you have succeeded in losing enough weight to have a scientifically healthy body you can now claim yourself to be a weight watcher.

Anyway, it is a fact that everything tend to go wrong during weight loss programs. The primary issue arises from the slowness of the overall process. Weight is not something that can be lost overnight. Often just shredding 10 pounds can take six months for some people. The lucky ones can do much faster than that with rigorous adherence to the program. Some of them can even shed 100 pounds or more in a year. However, the problem is it takes a lot of work to lose 2 pounds a week, every week, for a whole year and beyond. Only dieting usually would not do such a drastic job. It would definitely take a lot of workout, usually in the range of 1000 to 1500 calories burnt five days a week. The question is how long do you think you can continue to take such extraneous effort? Most people would quit in a month or two.

Majority of the people who are in it only to lose some weight would get tired probably in 3-4 months. Especially if they are not losing fast enough. And then there are times when people don't lose any weight, no matter what they do. Their bodies just hang on to every bit of mass. They are understandably the first group of people to lose confidence in it all. For the others who see little to moderate results may also get frustrated, bored and doubtful about the effectiveness of weight loss programs and slump into inactivity.

If you are one of them I do not blame you. I have thrown towel many times and I wasn't even trying to lose a lot. If you are at the other end of the spectrum where you must get rid of a good % of your body mass, your situation would get much worse than mine. At times you may even feel nothing was really working. You lost nothing or even worse, the wretched weight machine even showed a gain. You feel like dying. After all that hard work how was it even possible? *It happens to everybody.* Trust me. You need to memorize that statement and use it as a reminder that you are not alone and giving up was not an option. You need to get back and continue with it even though nothing seems to be working. Always remember the magic words

It happens to everybody.

The truth is - not everybody can cope up with the challenging times. Many easily give up. That's where comes your determination, mental strength and rationality.

If you are still ready to quit, give it one last thought. Quitting is easy. It is basically escaping the reality. Instead of completely quitting **how about just taking a break?**

A week's break should be fine, but no longer. By break I do mean break from all restrictions. Take it. It would definitely free your mind. But again,

Don't let it go for more than a week.

You want a break, not to break your commitment to the program. A week gives that nice length of rest without really disrupting your overall commitment. You allow that one week to roll into second week and it'll be months before you realize you have gained back most of what you had lost after plenty of hard work.

What can others do to ruin it for you?

That's the most unfortunate part of this endeavor. While others can do a lot to help you, they can also be equally effective in ruining it for you. And I am not saying it in a bad way. Often the people who love you the most may not share or understand your priorities. Sometimes they may even try to impose their priorities on you. They obviously want the best for you but may often inadvertently ignore your wishes.

I am sure we all have seen plenty of examples of that. From indulgent mother to loving uncle and aunts who all want to see you healthy and happy. The only problem is sometimes they do not necessarily have the eyes to see how you are suffering from all that attention. You often need a quiet corner, some silence to figure it all out in your mind. Sometimes it is hard to get. I guess those are the times when things do get challenging. All the stuff that you are trying to do – dieting, workouts, staying busy – takes a lot of effort, both physically and mentally. Often the physical part is much easier than handling it mentally. The pressure of it all can become overwhelming – the lure of going with your friends and family and have a calorie rich dinner, or to a drinking party...you can't really do that. At least you are trying hard not to do so. But how can you succeed if everybody is calling you...your phone ringing every few minutes. You are being told that it is okay to indulge sometimes. A little weight isn't going to kill you. However, all you really want to do is to eat a very light supper and watch a movie to forget about the hunger. It works for you. Only if everybody...the people who really love you...left you alone.

What I have just described can happen in many different ways and forms. Sometimes it can be your relatives or friends visiting you or vice versa. Some other times it can be a slew of different family events, parties after parties...you are with friends and family...everybody is happy, you are happy, life seems too broad to worry about some minor weight issue and soon you find yourself binging on food and/or alcohol. By the time all these madness ends – which can be weeks ...you are way off your schedule, your determination weakened, body slackened...you have literally become a mess.

It is really that easy to ruin everything.

When I say do it with *a smile* I don't mean you lose yourself in laughter. Smile is a symbolic gesture...*being at ease but not really relaxing or riding the wave.* You must avoid the scenarios I have just described. Don't allow yourself the indulgence to get into such uncontrolled overly happy and often carefree situation. I don't say you shouldn't participate or have visitors at your home or go visit your relatives, but do so with a lot of apprehension. Give your program the top priority, at least for several months, until you gain that strength which can guide you through just about any situation without having you to worry of losing control. With time you'll gain enough control to accompany your friends to a buffet and only eat what you find appropriate according to your program.

What can YOU do to ruin it?

The one single thing that you can do to ruin it all is:

Being Lazy

I realize it is not easy to follow the strenuous routine day after day, week after week. That's why I have tried to break things up; shown you way to do things in little pieces, without stressing yourself up too much. If you follow that you'll be able to continue steadily. You do too much you won't feel like doing it; you do too little, it won't work very well. Do just enough to keep going while feeling the effectiveness of it.

Feeling lazy is very humanly thing to do. I do not suggest you fight too hard when such laziness overpowers your normal life. *Sometimes giving in for a day or two may have a good impact*. But don't allow it go on for too long.

Taking things too easy

Okay, I asked you to take things easy. But do not overdo it. If you take it too easy then you would lose focus. Too much of anything is bad. Don't get too motivated and put all the good things in your life in jeopardy. At the same time, I repeat, nothing can be achieved without putting sufficient effort. Keep that in mind. You want to lose weight you must take some pain to do so. Just manage that pain. Don't at any point tell yourself *'if it doesn't work I'll try something else'*. That is a bad message to give to you. Remember within you there are several personalities – each with their own set of strength and weaknesses. You encourage the weakness all of them would make you weak. I know it is starting to sound like something taken from a psycho movie but by personality I simply mean different virtues of you. Sometimes you are very hard working; sometimes you are very laid back. Consider each of them as your one personality. You must ensure there is a good balance between them and one of them do not get an upper hand on the other one.

Listening to others when you shouldn't be

Okay, this is a strong statement to make. Listening to others cannot be bad all the time. We all have many well wishers who truly want us to succeed in life. Some of them may even be willing to go a long way to help us succeed. These are the people we should really value all through our lives. However, there are another set of people who are in a totally different spectrum. They may love you in their own way but may also have a tendency to insist you on doing things that are not in your best interest. These activities could be anything from partying to drinking to bungee jumping ... there's no limit. While it is greatly possible that you do like those activities as well but if they are coming between you and your target of weight loss you must make a choice. Do not at any point put weight loss at the back seat. It doesn't have to be on the driving seat but make it sit next to you, right on the passenger seat. Don't allow anybody to move you away from your goal. Remember, there are a lot of people out there who can try to convince you that all these weight loss stuff are complete crap and you look just beautiful as being overweight and you should be living your life to the fullest without going through such pain. Don't listen to them. Without getting any deeper into this scenario I want to remind you that you are here because you wanted to be here. You wanted to get healthy, fit and feel happier. Stay on the plan. However, I do not want you to be neglectful of your close friends. You need to manage them in a subtle way so that they realize that it is something that you really value and want to succeed. There is a great chance that they would start to play supportive roles. To put it concisely – ***unless you show some serious devotion others would not take it seriously***.

Chapter 10

How To Get Back On Track

Okay, so here's another very, very challenging thing to do. Let's say you were doing great, dieting, working out, losing (weight) steadily, feeling great about it all – and then something happened...something personal, family related, job related – there are so many things out there to spoil the day. So, as a result of that, you somehow got out of synch...and before you know you have turned into this couch potato, gained back more than what you had lost and the last thing you want to hear about is dieting, or workout or anything to do with that. And above all, you are not happy. You want to get back to the previous state but everything seems so hard, so impossible! And the problem is, the longer you wait to get back to your previous state the more desperate you become. Unfortunately that desperation does not always work for better future. Often it actually makes thing worse. It takes away the mental strength and replaces that with some sort of whim...fills you with opposing logic, tries to make you feel equally guilty and stubborn. This is a bad spot to be. You can't tolerate it and you can't get out of it. What do you do now? How to get out of this situation as a winner?

It is not easy!

I know you already know this but nevertheless I would go ahead and spell it out. **It does happen to real people and it is very hard to snap out of it.**

How can that help you? By making you feel human. Often such simple things can provide strong moral boost. Just knowing that you are not alone can be, though strangely, empowering.

Do the following and you should be able to start all over again.

1. Start with some sort of meditation. This can very well be religious chores, simple yoga or other similar procedures or systems. This would work on to provide you some sort of focus. Here I must

mention I do not encourage people to choose one over the other. Simply go for what works better for you. While I am not much of a religious person from my experience I have noticed it works magic for the true believers. Anyway, there are plenty of options to choose from.

2. Another good way to get into the mood is to stay away from social gatherings for a little while, especially the type where there are lots of food and drink. Big parties often make people carefree which in turn may encourage consuming disproportionate amount of food and liquor. That simply won't help.

3. If you do first and second items of this list you'll eventually get back your focus and will be ready to start over. Remember the two guiding forces: **focus and manage**. It's not easy by any means but it is doable.

4. It is a fact that burning calories while playing a sport is a more preferred way to remain healthy. Find a sport that you like. Try to play it a few hours a week. If you need a partner find one. Play lightly in the beginning. Enjoy the game. Couple of weeks

would make you fitter. In third or fourth week you'll even be able to get on to a cardio vascular machine. Make no mistake, if you can lose all your calories from playing sports that is definitely great. However, for muscle building certain type of equipment is needed. So, at some point you may have to visit the gym or buy some weights to do it at home.

5. Once you have gotten back to the sports/workout cycle only then slowly introduce dieting. Don't try to leap. Do a little bit at a time. Don't go for Atkin's meat based diet. Simply resort to balanced diet. Eat slightly less than normal. Eat everything you used to eat, just in lesser quantity. Even better if you can reduce the fat quantity. Reduce your daily intake by two hundred calories or so in the first week. In the following week by 300 calories. Go on slowly until you start to feel stressed. Here you stop. There's no need for you to be stressed. Slow and steady does win the race when it comes to weight loss.

6. Couple up with a friend, colleague, or relative with similar weight loss interest– whoever you can find.

Having a partner can be one of the best things to provide motivation. Often each other becomes the driving force to keep things going.

7. Create a plan; itemize things that you need to do to get back on. Being able to identify the required steps and time stamp them is always a very positive step forward as it works in clearing up people's mind and give you a much needed focus and motivation.

And of course, **apply your will power. This is really about you. You are the hero of this story. You must act.**

Chapter 11

Maintaining

Most Important phase

This is probably the most important phase in this whole procedure. Very often people can come up with enough mental strength and driving force to go through all the trouble to lose some weight (rarely people lose all the weight that they had planned for) but then when it comes to maintianing what was achieved things start to get in the wrong side of the road. This is a common phenomena. People takes great effort to lose weight but very few succeeds in keeping it that way. This may happen due to many reasons but very often simple things are more than enough to disrupt and destroy hard fought achievements. Things that took years to gain are lost just in a month. That's how we are...most of us are. Like it or not.

When we want we can do incredible things but then we are also very much capable of destroying it all – whether in whim or being drawn into unfavorable situations – that can be anybody's guess. But the truth probably is somewhere in the middle. That is why my suggestion is simple:

Once you have achieved your goal or a partial success, the only target should become '**no going back**'. However, it is easy to say than doing. That's why for most people it is important to actually come up with a strategy to handle this. Let's see what type of strategy might help us handle it in the long term – we are thinking in months and years and not in weeks.

So, if you have gained a few pounds back because you attended couple of big parties and gobbled up lots of food (oh well, who are we fooling? It defintiely takes much more than that!) – what to do now? Not to worry. You are covered in our **universal strategy** – something that ought to work for everybody because it is hardly a strategy. It is more like alligning ourselves to our basic self and slowly guiding ourselves to the right path. What is that right path?

The Wave

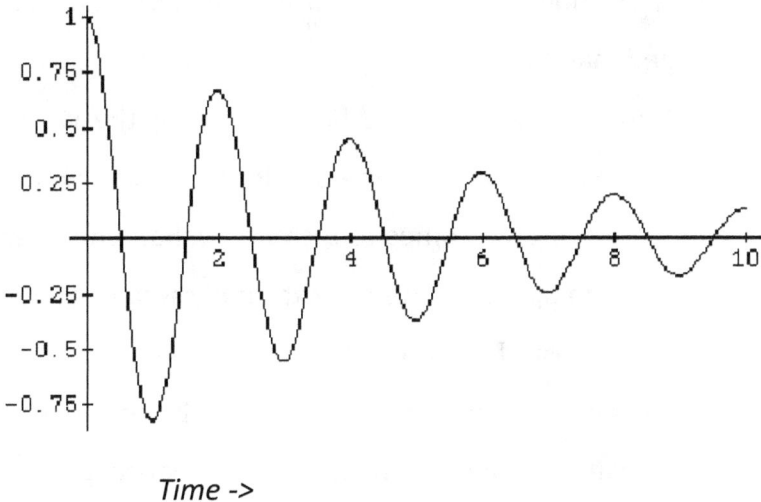

Time ->

A wave that starts with high *y* value but slowly decreases – coming closer to the center over time

You may be looking at that wavy image and wondering what am I suggesting you do? Nothing really. However, before I explain what is my '*nothing*' let me explain what this graph really means.

Most people who try to lose weight goes through many phases, some of these phases are quite repetitive. They would usually be able to reduce some weight but then end up gaining it back. Sometime later they usually get back into it again and repeat the same cycle. With every repetition they continue to get better. Eventually if they stay at it long enough they succeed in losing enough weight and maintaining it.

Now let's consider the first section of the wave. The down slope can be considered as losing weight, which at some point of time comes to a complete halt and over time start to go up, unless we are extremely serious about maintaining. Most of us aren't. As a result we start to gain back, represented by the rise. The peak can be considered as the worst situation. From here a conscience person usually can get back to the program and the wave repeats, possibly with longer amplitude (duration in our case).

Let's talk about the worst situation. At this point you are eating more, feeling lazy, not doing any workouts, clearly gaining weight and are terrified to stand on the scale. All of these are terrible things.

Or are they? May be not as bad as we think. As I have mentioned this is usually the point where most people bounce back. If anybody allows sliding beyond this point then they may enter a region from where there is no return. That is rather unusual and scarce and I would not discuss that here.

Now, let me tell you this - *do not feel bad about your lapses*. It is, believe it or not, the most common thing that all aspiring *weight losers* experience. It is quite normal and in a way not so bad because it tests your determination and willingness. It also give you an opportunity to prove yourself to you. *If you have done it once you can defintiely do it again*. Now to provide a few words of encouragement:

- It is easy to say *'let's start over'* than to actually do it. Even before you plan to restart make sure the followings are true:
  - You enjoy the process
  - You are smiling because you have nothing to lose but weight
  - You are determined enough to hit another high point (losing as much weight as you can in one attempt)
- Trust me next time the wave will be smaller. Things would get better.

Food:

As you ride the waves and slide back into the valleys you would for sure figure out what type of food working for you and what not. We can do a lot of researches, experiements and analysis but at the end each one of us have a different body, different set of criteria that governs our rate of burn or metabolism and appetite for food. It has been my observation that each individual eventually need to find out the following three things about his/her food choices:

1. What mix of protein, carbo and fat worked the best. Don't forget carbo includes vegetables and fruits as well. It is better not to be on fruits too much.

2. How many meals and snacks work out the best? The timing of each meal and snack may be important too as they may form a habitual trend for you. You miss the rythm everything may just fall off.

3. How to manage the cravings? In the beginning this could become the major concern but eventually as you get into the cycle of ups and

downs for a couple of times you simply would figure out exactly what works for you to curb your cravings for certain type of foods. For many this could be sweets, for others it could be fatty, fried food. Believe me you can definitely win over such cravings but it does need a good amount of mental strength and some help from family and friends. Just in case you are having issues with it do this simple trick – do not see, smell or hear about them. That's why I said you need help from your family and friends. Most are very willing to help out. If necessary don't be shy to spell it out to the people who are around you.

Workout:

This is often the key to returning to the program. Usually just reducing food intake never do the trick. It would only keep you hungry and remind you all the time that you are in that stupid dieting thing again. Such thought is serously damaging. That's why it is important to give the process a somewhat different texture to make it look and feel more interesting. And that is what *workout* does. It makes the process not just bearable but even enjoyble when done properly. Why? Because now you are not just dieting or starving to lose a few pounds but you are actually trying to get fit. That's a complete different ball game. Getting fit – provides a different perspective. It sounds good, and fun. After all it is almost synonym to sports – something that we like so much, more or less.

So, the question now is, have you figured out what kind of workout works the best for you? I had suggested that when you first start the program - go slow. However, once you get used to it your body can definitely take more, considering you have been continuing with the workout routine at least two three days a week.

Remember we are now talking about your second or third time into this. Obviously you are back here because you kind of failed to sustain your success for long. Something almost everybody is guilty of. No need to feel guilty or sad. Just enjoy the ride. If at some point you slump, you slump. Rise back. That's the magic phrase – **Rise back**.

<u>If you have done it once you can do it again.</u>

Other habits:

Remember that your goal is not only to lose weight. Alone it would not work, at least not to the level I am trying to take you to. If you are a smoker, a drinker or have other addictive habits than perhaps this is the right time and opportunity to work on all of them together. Your mind is strong, determination high and body is getting stronger and tougher – what time could be better to enslave your own bad habits and simply say good bye to them. Take this opportunity to put everything in your life in a straight path, as much possible, you'll feel like a million dollar person. If I even start blabbering about how proud and strong I feel for quitting my smoking habit many years ago after smoking for very long time starting as early as twelve you may not be able to stop me. I can only say briefly – the feeling is overwhelming. It gives me the kind of pleasure that somebody can get, just to give an analogy, climbing the Everest. Both seem impossible at one point but yet so many have done it. I am out of smoking for 19 years now. I consider that one of my biggest achievements.

Anyway, what I was trying to say is – once you are in the mood utilize it as much as you can. Hopefully you'll emerge as a better person and not necessarily just leaner. If not, what to lose? It's really a win-win situation.

Chapter 12

Stay Alert

Don't let yourself slip – not totally

Let's say you have ridden through the waves and finally you have made it. By making it I mean you have not only reached your target, you have also successfully taught yourself to live within a boundary allowing you to stay in a relatively enjoyable and acceptable condition. It is quite doable. It is also quite easy to fail. There are people on both ends. The magic to that long term success is simple – *make it become your natural life style and not an imposed one.*

You enjoy food, no worries. You do not need to sacrifice anything but the portions. Instead of three pieces of roasted chicken perhaps eat one but eat it slowly relishing every bit of it. Really, at the end two things are happening. One, your mouth is enjoying the taste of it, two – your belly is starting to get filled. After dieting or controlling your food intake for a while your stomach would start to shrink for sure. There won't be the need of too much food to have that nice feeling of being full any more. However your greed for food may still be very much alive. So, all you need to do is to teach yourself to *eat slowly* - <u>*chew longer, wait before taking the next mouthful, make an effort to enjoy the food to its end*</u>.

If your life has taken a bad turn and suddenly you do not feel like caring for anything – good or bad – it is greatly possible that you'll start to eat a lot and even abuse substances. I can't say how far you may go with it but one thing I want to add that everybody goes through such time of depression. Even when you are going through a bad patch remind yourself the moments of pride, the strength that you displayed months after months, the control you showed days after days – it works. May be not the first time but it would work. Just don't allow yourself to be totally driven away. **Give yourself a chance to fight back**.

You may also end up going through a time when things start to get too good, life become a full time party, too many friends, too many dinner invitations etc. etc. Often such times do worse than the down times. Why? This is how I explain it: you start to get driven away by a sense of success which works on to change your perception of good and bad. Being fit or lean may not be as important as you thought it were. After all there are tons of obese and successful people out there. Who cares?

Don't allow yourself to get to that point. Success is good but it needn't play a role to change you at the core. Keep your values. With good health your happiness can only go up. Don't let it slip at any cost. Make time to spend half an hour doing some workout every other day in the least, keep alive the calorie counter that you have established in your mind. Don't let it go. It is your friend - *in happiness and in sorrow.*

And then there are those trips - joy trips, business trips, travels; people tend to lose their guards during these trips. It become a *let's just have a little fun* type thing. But besides increasing the gut size what primarily such lapses do is that they take away *the hard earned attitude toward good health.* Nothing is easy on this Earth. You let go your determination and allow yourself to become mellow about something that requires maximum determination it is going to be a while before you can snap out of it.

Worthless logic

Often I have heard people saying that some people ate so much but still were so thin. The suggestion here is that the difference in metabolism is so big that one person is gaining weight just by eating little food while some others, the lucky ones with huge metabolism, gained nothing even after gorging on food.

The above is a misinformed perception. Yes, metabolism can make some difference. However, it won't be that noticeable. Remember, a large person inherently have higher metabolism because of the body mass. So, if you see a slim person who seems to eat a lot be sure that s/he may have issues with indigestion, may be extremely active, or could be simply rationing her diet other times when s/he is not in public eyes.

Don't allow yourself to even indulge on such worthless perception. It usually does the bad. Our bodies are our tools. Not the other way around. A tool does what the user wants it to do.

If, for whatever reason, you simply can't force yourself back to the program for a while, don't beat yourself up over this. If possible simply get away from your regular life style for a little while. Take a break from all of it – I might dare to say. Come back with twice the eagerness and strength. No bullshit, no hopeless sighs, no worthless rationalization. It is a beast and you must fight it. That's the only way to win here.

Chapter 13

Myths

We all, more or less, heard or believe in things that do not necessarily have a lot to hold ground. Often such things can misguide us, shift us from our goals, and make things more complicated and harder. It doesn't have to be like that. Know about the myths of weight loss and make educated decisions.

Myth: Carbohydrate causes weight gain

Before exploring the impact of carbohydrate on weight loss we should spend a little time on understanding what Carbohydrate is as it is probably one of the most talked about topics when it comes to weight loss.

Carbohydrates – what is it?

Carbohydrates are compounds used by our bodies to create energy. Almost everything we eat has some kind of carbohydrate – in various forms and different amounts. All carbohydrates are made up sugar molecules working as building blocks. The sugar that we eat in our food is one of the most basic carbohydrates consisting of only a handful of these building blocks. Other more starchy or complex carbohydrates are found in rice, bread, pasta etc.

Fiber, classed as a carbohydrate, has a different set of functions which are very important for our body functions.

Carbohydrates – why do we need it?

Carbohydrates are source of energy for us. We use them to keep our bodies active and our vital internal organs working properly. The process is simple: we eat carbohydrate -> digestive system breaks it down into simple sugars, such as glucose –> glucose is then circulated in the blood and takes it to every cell in the body.

If we do not eat enough carbohydrate our body will break down fat and protein to get the required glucose. Protein is important for our body and has a different set of functions like growing, repairing and not a preferred source of energy. So, unless we have a large amount of stored fat in our body it is important to intake sufficient Carbohydrates.

What type of Carbohydrate to eat

Yes, considering your situation there can be something called good carb and bad carb. You must have heard these terms many times already.

Before discussing that lets briefly touch one point – generally while carbohydrates are our energy source too much of it can be bad as the excess gets converted in fat which in turn causes weight gain. So, it is greatly possible that when eaten without proper knowledge and quantity it can contribute in an unfavorable way if you are weight conscious. That's why having proper knowledge and taking effort to figure out the right quantity and sticking to it is important. The problem is not with carbohydrate, it is really with us.

So, what is good carbo and what is bad carbo?

Let's take a quick look at them.

Bad carbo

Sugary foods, such as cokes, cookies, cakes etc. contains high amount of sugar and may also contain very high amount of fat and beside providing a good sugar kick has little beneficial nutrients. They are also bad for tooth if proper care is not taken to clean mouth after eating them. While they do provide lots of energy, they also create an issue of overeating. This happens for two reasons. First of all, most of us like sugary food. Secondly when a certain food contains a lot of calorie in a small portion we often do not feel full or content and end up eating large portion. The end result is too much calories consumed.

Good carbo

As we have found out a little earlier that we do need to eat necessary amount of carbohydrate from starchy food like rice, wheat etc. From recent studies it is found that whole grain foods contains fiber and other useful nutrients which gets removed when grains are refined to give it the whiter look.

Another interesting thing about whole grains is that they generally take longer to get digested. This in turn may provide the sense of being full for longer and make it easier to control the urge for eating.

Beside that fruits, vegetables are also source of good carbohydrates generally.

How much carbohydrate do I need?

Most dieticians believe that most of the energy that we need for our daily life should come from carbohydrates, preferably good carbohydrates so that we get not only the energy we need but also the extra nutritional stuff like fiber, vitamins as well. There may be slightly different numbers hovering around but generally 40-50% should come from carbohydrate, preferably majority of it from whole grains or less sugary foods. Normally it is not a problem as we already enjoy starchy foods. The issue is really to pick the right type in right amount. Calorie counting is important here.

So, is it a myth or true that carbohydrate causes weight gain?

We know by now that it can only be true if you are not paying attention to what type of carbo you are eating and of what amount. According to a study published in April 2012, participants who ate a low-calorie diet high in whole wheat for 12 weeks lost more fat than a group that ate a low-cal diet high in refined wheat, most likely because the extra fiber in whole grains was more filling.

Myth: Add longer workouts

This is a very common and interesting topic. We all know workout is good for overall health and to lose weight, when done properly. I have discussed that as well in details. Now the question is if we increase the workout resulting into more calorie burn would it be good for weight loss?

Many people may think it would as we are essentially burning more calories and possibly more fat. Unfortunately weight loss is not always a simple equation of burning calories or fat calories. There are other factors involved, primarily concerning food intake. In a recent Danish study published in September 2012 found that one group of overweight participants that did only 30 minutes of workout as oppose to the other group that did 60 minutes had lost more weight during the 13-week study. How is that possible? I think we all must have already guessed the answer. When you are working out more you do burn more calories but at the same time you are also creating higher appetite for food. As a result at the end of the day you may end up eating more calories than you had burnt during the extra workout.

Of course if you can do extra workout and force yourself to maintain exact same diet as before you'll lose more. Unfortunately that is hard and rarely happens.

Final words on this: don't go overboard. Make sure whatever you do that does not have any major impact on your overall amount of food intake. In weight loss program the most important factor is food. Workout is complementary.

Myth: No desserts

Many people are really sweet lovers. It is generally true that most sweets or desserts are heavy on calories and sugar. None of it is very good for us under normal circumstances. It is reasonable to think that for a weight loss program to succeed keeping the sweet intake very low is mandatory, even better if we can totally get rid of it.

However, it doesn't necessarily support the reality. Again, it is a matter of balancing between calories, nutrition and food preferences. If you are eating a piece of cake that contains 500 calories then you'll have to compensate for that by cutting calorie intakes coming from other type of foods. Let's say you are on an 1800 calorie diet. You need to ensure that you get all the nutrition your body requires within that. A piece of cake has a lot of deliciousness but little nutrition. So, a better balance can be reached by eating a smaller portion worth 250 calories. It should still be enough to provide you that much enjoyed sugary kick. The good? Now you have an extra 250 calories to fill in with more nutritional food. According to a study published in March 2012 in the journal Steroids: Researchers found that participants who ate a 600-calorie, carb- and protein-rich breakfast that included dessert, such as chocolate or ice cream, lost more weight over four months (and kept more off the following four months) than a group that ate a low-carb morning meal.

Myth: Don't eat any fat at all

When we are trying to lose weight one of the things that we read about the most is definitely *fat*. No wonder why. This is what we are out to get rid of. We know it is bad, tends to get stored in our body for long time, make us look big, chubby and unhealthy. The more we can keep this evil away from our diet the better.

However, we have to be careful on that approach. Our bodies need fat for all kind of reason. It is generally accepted that 30% of our daily calorie need should come from fatty food. How does that help? In a study published in the Journal of the American Medical Association, researchers compared participants on three diets—low-fat, low-glycemic (carbohydrate-rich foods that do not raise blood sugar levels too much compared to glucose), and low-carb. Eating a low-fat diet decreased resting energy expenditure (or the number of calories you burn at rest) the most. Cutting back on fat also affected hormones essential to keeping cholesterol and insulin in check.

So, summarily it can be said that we should be eating some fat as part of our diet. If not then the body may start to eat up from muscle. Better to take unsaturated fat which are considered healthy fat like oil, fish fat, nuts etc.

Myth: Zero-calorie sweeteners are best remedy

Anybody who loves regular soda and sweets or desserts would definitely appreciate the fact that zero calorie sweeteners provide a good option to be able to drink or eat the same stuff without the calories and sometimes not even sacrificing the taste that much. The choices for zero calorie sweeteners sucralose, aspartame, and stevia are appealing but we need to be careful on that approach as well. According to a joint study statement by the American Heart Association and the American Diabetes Association, the scientific evidence connecting zero-calorie sweeteners with long-term weight loss is inconclusive. Why? One of the main problems is overcompensation. If you save 150 calories by drinking a diet soda, and then reward yourself with an extra helping at dinner, you've negated any calorie-saving benefit.

So, generally speaking, using sweeteners are not bad, especially knowing that there has not been any study showing any harmful Impact of them on human body when used in safe quantity. However, the allowable amount is usually very little. Let me provide an example. For Equals it is about six small packs a day. A diet soda usually contains about that much.

Appendix A

Metabolism

What is it?

How many times have I heard people blaming slow metabolism for being overweight? Many, many times. Does that actually stand any ground? Let's see if it does. Often people talks about metabolism either not exactly knowing what it means or knowing only partially. So, it would definitely help exploring the true definition of it.

There are lots of definitions out there. All says the same thing but in different ways. Some are easy to grasp some are more technical in nature. I would resort to the easy one.

Our body needs energy to run. We eat food and drinks to provide it the raw material. The food gets processed generating energy. The procedure or process that allows the body to convert the food into energy is called metabolism. It is a complex process, at the end of which body receives energy that it can then use to function.

Basal metabolism: This is really what we refer to as our metabolism. This is the energy that our body uses to run our essential body functions like breathing, blood circulation, growth, repair etc. Regardless of our physical activities this is the calories continues to be spent by the body. This is what is truly our metabolism is. The BMR or Basal Metabolism rate is also expressed as the amount of energy spent by human and animals at rest. There are calculators to calculate the BMR based on age, weight and activity.

Basal metabolism accounts for most of the energy that we spend in a whole day, in the range of 70-80%.

What about the rest?

Two other processes also are responsible for burning calories.

- **Food processing** (thermogenesis): The food we consume gets digested, absorbed, transported etc. and in the process spent some energy as well. This accounts about 10% of the total calories that we consume. It is mentionable here that specific type of food takes more energy to get processed such as protein burns more calories than carbohydrate.

- **Physical activity**: This is really the icing at the top of a cake. Basal metabolism and thermogenesis are responsible for 80% of all the calories we burn. The rest is burnt during any activities that we do all through the day including sports, exercises and other activities that create physical exertion. If we do a lot of workout or our job requires hard physical work then at the end of the day we'll be spending much more at the top of our basal metabolism.

Metabolism and weight

Coming back to the most interesting topic regarding weight loss. Is it possible that some people has very high metabolic rate and no matter how much they eat their body simply gobbles up all the energy and keep them in great shape while some others no matter how little they eat continues to grow big? Definitely not.

As we have already explored about the metabolism we know that this is the calorie we all burn without even doing anything. However, we definitely do not burn same amount. It would depend on our age, weight and life style to some extent. To put it even more clearly, a skinny person has a lower metabolism than an overweight person, generally speaking. At the top of that as long as we remain active we'll continue to burn extra calories. Often, skinny people are very physically active, burning big amount of calories every day. This is where an overweight person may fall behind. With excessive weight comes inconvenience in movement. People often get lazy and even mild physical activities can become painful and stressful. When such situation persist an overweight person continue to gain more. The problem is never with metabolism, but with the individuals who cannot remain sufficiently physically active. .

Clearly, blaming the metabolism rate as being poor or low is useless and far from truth. It would not help anybody and only provide with an excuse that is not really a cause for weight gain.

How to enhance metabolism?

We really have little control over our basal metabolic rate. It does decrease over age and may be controlled slightly by choosing food and activities but beside that there really not much room to manipulate. As we have already discussed this before, protein takes more energy to get digested and absorbed. Hence eating more protein may cause metabolism to go slightly up but that may not have a better effect on the body in the long run. Also, having more muscle automatically increase basal metabolism because body spent more energy to keep them energized than it does to other type of cells. So, by being active and by building extra muscles we can help our metabolism to go up. A general idea is that every pound of extra muscle can burn 50 extra calories just for maintenance.

The best way to enhance metabolism, not the basal metabolism alone, but the overall metabolism or the energy spent in a whole day is to consider the complete picture.

Now, not all activities burn fat equally if weight loss is your goal. It is important to pick appropriate activities based on individual preference. Aerobic exercises are considered efficient way to burn more calories. It includes walking, swimming, bicycling etc. Keeping the heart rate at 120 beats per sec is the optimal condition for maximizing fat burn. So, whatever exercise we do it is important to control the exertion and allow the heart to reach and stay around that. Too quick heart rate would pull in carbohydrate or glucose to meet the immediate need of the body and won't burn as much fat. It is suggested that performing 30 minutes of aerobic exercise on regular basis would probably see best result.

Using weights to build muscles is also a good way to burn calories though by nature it works quite differently than aerobic exercise. Weight lifting is considered heavy exercise and cannot be done on regular basis. Twice a week probably is best which allows the muscles to repair all the tears that happen during a session. Also, initially it burns much less calorie within a session but when performed for longer duration it may burn just as much calories as in an aerobic session. However, I would not advice this type of exercise for everybody. There is a good amount of risk of getting hurt or over stressing the muscles. Injuries may happen and usually do not heal quickly which may take away the pace of progress and put a person behind plan. However, doing light weights is good for most people.

Metabolism related diseases

A metabolic disorder occurs when abnormal chemical reactions in your body disrupt this process. When this happens, you might have too much of some substances or too little of other ones that you need to stay healthy.

You can develop a metabolic disorder when some organs, such as your liver or pancreas, become diseased or do not function normally. Diabetes is an example.

There are many diseases that are categorized as metabolism related and we would not try to explain them here.

Appendix B

Calculation of daily calorie need

The first step to any weight loss program should be determining daily calorie need. As we have described in the book all of our activities must be carefully planned and guided by this number.

There are several different parts of calculating overall calorie requirement in a full day.

Basal metabolism

First is to calculate the BMR or basal metabolic rate or the energy used by our bodies during rest. The formula uses metric measurements (1 inch - 2.54 cm and 1 kilogram = 2.2 lbs). For men, the formula is:

BMR = 66 + (13.7 X wt in kg) + (5 X ht in cm) - (6.8 X age in years)

From this formula it is clearly visible that over age BMR would decrease while a person's weight and height would play a role to increase it.

Let's consider two men, one young and average height and weight, the other one tall and heavier but older.

150 pounds = 68 kg; age = 20; height = 175 cm (5'9")

BMR = 66 + (13.7 X 68) + (5 x 175) – (6.8 x 20)

BMR = 66 + 931.6 + 875 - 136 = 1736.6 calories per day

Therefore, if a 185 lb man is 6 feet tall (72 inches) and 35 years old, you would compute his BMR by substituting the numbers:

185 pounds = 84 kg; age = 35; height = 183 cm (6')

BMR = 66 + (13.7 X 84) + (5 x 183) – (6.8 x 35)

BMR = 66 + 1152 + 915 - 238 = 1895 calories per day

The difference in BMR is only about 150 calories per day. This is not considerably much if you think in terms of food. A loaf of whole grain bread is 120 calories.

Let's see how this works out for women.

The formula for a woman's BMR is:

BMR = 655 + (9.6 X wt in kg) + (1.8 X ht in cm) - (4.7 X age in years)

If a woman is 130 lbs., 63 inches tall and 35 years of age, use the following calculation:

BMR = 655 + (9.6 x 59) + (1.8 x 160) - (4.7 x 35)

BMR = 655 + (566.4) + (288) - (164.5) = 1344.9 calories per day

If a woman is 160 lbs., 65 inches tall and 20 years of age, use the following calculation:

BMR = 655 + (9.6 x 72.72) + (1.8 x 165) - (4.7 x 20)

BMR = 1556 calories per day

The difference comes up to 220 calories or couple of whole grain bread loaves. The point that can easily be made from these calculations is that just because you are big doesn't mean your calorie requirement would be much higher than the person who looks like just a fraction of you unless you are physically extremely active. That's coming next.

Consider physical activity level:

Multiply the BMR using the Harris Benedict equation (details below), estimating your approximate activity level:

Sedentary (little or no exercise) = BMR x 1.2;

Lightly active (light exercise or sports 1 to 3 days per week) = BMR x 1.375;

Moderately active (moderate exercise or sports 3 to 5 days per week) = BMR x 1.55;

Very active (hard exercise or sports 6 to 7 days a week) = BMR x 1.725 and

If you are extra active (very hard exercise or sports with a physical job) = BMR x 1.9

Harris Benedict Equation

The **Harris Benedict Equation** is a formula that uses the BMR and then applies an activity factor to determine the total daily energy expenditure (calories) of an individual.

However, it omits the lean body mass factor. Note that leaner bodies need more calories than less leaner ones due to higher quantity of muscles. Therefore, this equation is less accurate for individuals who are either very muscular or very much overweight.

Body mass index (BMI) is a measure of body fat based on height and weight that applies to adult men and women. BMI calculators are easily available on the web and the scores may provide good indication of weight related issues if exist.

English BMI Formula

BMI = (Weight in Pounds / (Height in inches x Height in inches)) x 703

Metric BMI Formula

BMI = (Weight in Kilograms / (Height in Meters x Height in Meters))

BMI Categories:

Use the following categories to determine where you belong. This can help you to determine how much weight you should be losing if any.

Underweight = <18.5

Normal weight = 18.5–24.9

Overweight = 25–29.9

Obesity = BMI of 30 or greater

Appendix C

Some possible snacks

So what qualifies as a snack?

The answer may vary person to person. Some people may consider a piece of cake to be a snack. Some others may consider a few pieces of baby carrots a snack. It doesn't take much to see the huge difference in the two snacks – in calorie content and nutrition. A piece of cake even when sugar free has several hundred calories while a few pieces of baby carrots with some sort of dip couldn't be more than fifty calories. Now consider how many of these snacks you think you want to eat everyday in between meals? Two is probably the standard answer. One between breakfast and lunch; one between lunch and supper.

It is important to ensure that the snacks do not consist of too much calories and by no means turns into a meal. A snack should be less or equal to a hundred calories when you are in weight loss mode. At most 150 but not a calorie more unless you are working out hard, which if you remember I had advised against.

Okay, so let's check out a possible list of snacks. The following list is a compilation of information that is available on the web. I present it here simply to educate you and to help you determine some healthy and low calorie choices for snacks. Not all can be appealing to everybody. Pick what you like and rotate as it seems appropriate.

#	Prep name	Details
Sweet		
1	Mini PB&F	One fig Newton with 1 teaspoon peanut butter
2	Chocolate Banana	Half a frozen banana dipped in two squares of melted dark chocolate.
3	Frozen grapes (any color)	1 cup (about 28 grapes), stuck in the freezer for 2+ hours.
4	Honeyed Yogurt	: ½ cup nonfat Greek yogurt with a dash of cinnamon and 1 teaspoon honey.
5	Spiced Orange	One orange— about the size of a tennis ball— sprinkled with cinnamon.
6	Grilled Pineapple	2 ¼-inch thick pineapple rounds (about 1 cup), grilled (or sautéed)

		for two minutes or until golden.
7	Berries n' Cream	1 cup blueberries with 2 tablespoons whipped topping.
8	Stuffed Figs	Two small dried figs with 1 tablespoon reduced-fat ricotta stuffed inside. Sprinkle with cinnamon.
9	Oats n' Berries	⅓ cup rolled oats (cooked with water), topped with cinnamon and ¼ cup fresh berries.
10	Dark Chocolate	One block, or three squares.
11	Nut-Stuffed Date	One Medjool Date filled with one teaspoon natural unsalted almond butter.
12	Chocolate Milk	6 ounces skim milk mixed with 2 teaspoons chocolate syrup.
13	Cinnamon Applesauce	1 cup unsweetened applesauce. Or, try this homemade version!
14	Citrus-Berry Salad	1 cup mixed berry salad (raspberries, strawberries, blueberries, and/or blackberries) tossed with one tablespoon fresh-squeezed orange juice.
15	Maple-Pumpkin Yogurt	½ cup non-fat regular yogurt (go Greek for extra protein!) with 2 tablespoons pumpkin puree and 1 teaspoon maple syrup.
16	Chocolate Pudding	One 4oz package. Try a fat/sugar free version or a homemade one!
17	Chocolate Covered	Five strawberries dipped in two squares melted dark chocolate.

	Strawberries	
18	Vanilla and Banana Smoothie	½ cup sliced banana, ¼ cup nonfat vanilla yogurt, and a handful of ice blended until smooth.
19	MYO Banana Chips	One sliced banana dipped in lemon juice and baked.
20	Baked Apple	One tennis ball-sized apple, cored, filled with 1 teaspoon brown sugar and cinnamon, and baked until tender.
21	Fruity Waffles	One 7-grain frozen waffle toasted and topped with ¼ cup fresh mixed berries.
22	Skinny S'more	Two graham crackers with one roasted marshmallow and one small square dark chocolate.
23	Cinnamon Graham Crackers & Peanut butter	Two graham cracker squares with 1 teaspoon peanut butter and a sprinkle of cinnamon.
24	Cereal and Milk	½ cup rice krispies with ½ cup skim milk.
25	Milk n' Cookies	Five animal crackers with ½ cup skim milk.
26	Warm Spiced Cider	6 ounces apple cider with sprinkles of cinnamon and nutmeg, warmed.
27	Citrus Sherbet	½ cup lime sherbet (about one standard-sized ice-cream scoop) with ½ sliced kiwi.
28	Jelly Beans	25 of 'em! Although we don't

			recommend these.
29	Tropical Juice Smoothie		¼ cup pineapple juice, orange juice, and apple juice, blended with ice.
30	Café Latte		8 ounces steamed skim milk with 1 shot espresso.
31	Marshmallow Pear		½ pear diced and topped with 1 tablespoon marshmallow fluff.
32	Protein Shake		One scoop protein powder with 8 ounces water (choose from tasty powder flavors like cookies n' cream and chocolate peanut butter!).
33	M.Y.O. Popsicle		8 ounces lemonade frozen in an ice pop mold, or use a small paper cup as a mold.
34	Apple Chips		Munch on ¾ cup of kinds like these, or use this recipe! Savory Satisfaction
35	Carrots n' Hummus		About 10 baby carrots with 2 tablespoons hummus.
36	Pistachios		A couple handfuls— about 25 nuts (Crackin' them open will take more time and avoid grabbing 25 more).
37	Cheese n' Crackers		Five Kashi 7-grain crackers with 1 stick reduced-fat string cheese.
38	Dippy Egg		One over easy egg with ½ slice whole-wheat toast, sliced (to dip in yolk!).
39	Cheesy Breaded		Two roasted plum tomatoes sliced and topped with 2 tablespoons

	Tomatoes	breadcrumbs and a sprinkle of parmesan cheese.
40	Curried Sweet Potato	One medium sweet potato (about 5 inches long) cooked for six minutes in the microwave and mashed with 1 teaspoon curry, and a sprinkle of salt and pepper.
41	"Cheesy" Popcorn	2 cups air-popped popcorn with 1 tablespoon nutritional yeast— it'll taste like real cheese!
42	Guacamole stuffed Egg Whites	Halve a hardboiled egg, remove yolk, and stuff the empty space with 2 tablespoons guacamole (avocado, lime, cilantro and salt).
43	Grilled Spinach and Feta Polenta	3 oz polenta (about the size of a deck of cards) cooked with 1 ½ cups water and topped with 1 teaspoon feta cheese and a handful spinach.
44	Soy Edamame	¼ cup boiled Edamame with 1 teaspoon soy sauce.
45	Dijon Pretzels	Two pretzel rods with 1 tablespoon Dijon mustard.
46	Crunchy Curried Tuna Salad	½ cup canned tuna with 1 teaspoon curry powder, 1 tablespoon chopped red onion, and two ribs celery (chopped).
47	Greek Tomatoes	One tomato (about the size of a tennis ball) chopped and mixed with 1 tablespoon feta and a squeeze of lemon juice.
48	Shrimp	Eight medium sized shrimp boiled

	Cocktail	and served with 2 tablespoons classic cocktail sauce.
49	Smoked Beef Jerky	About 1 ounce— look for low sodium versions!
50	Cheddar and Tomato Soup	½ cup tomato soup with 1 tablespoon shredded low-fat cheddar cheese.
51	Kale Chips	½ cup raw kale— stems removed— baked with 1 teaspoon olive oil at 400° until crisp.
52	Sweet Potato Fries	One light-bulb sized sweet potato sliced, tossed with 1 teaspoon olive oil, and baked at 400° for 10 minutes.
53	Cucumber Sandwich	½ English muffin with 2 tablespoons cottage cheese and three slices of cucumber.
54	Mixed Olives	About 8 olives.
55	Antipasto Plate	One Pepperocini, a ½ inch cube of cheddar cheese, one slice pepperoni, and one olive.
56	Pumpkin Seeds	2 tablespoons pumpkin seeds, sprayed with oil (just a spritz!) and baked at for 400° for 15 minutes or until brown. Sprinkle with kosher salt.
57	Choco-Soy Nuts	3 tablespoons soy nuts with 1 teaspoon cocoa nibs.
58	Wasabi Peas	About ⅓ cup of these green treats.
59	Cheesy Roasted Asparagus	Four spears (spritzed with olive-oil spray) and topped with 2 tablespoons grated parmesan

		cheese, baked for 10 minutes at 400°.
60	Cucumber salad	One large cucumber (sliced) with 2 tablespoons chopped red onion and 2 tablespoons apple-cider vinegar.
61	Spinach and Feta Egg-White Scramble	Three egg whites scrambled and mixed with ½ cup raw spinach and 1 tbsp feta cheese. Cook in frying pan or zap in microwave until egg whites are no longer runny (about 1-2 minutes).
62	Crunchy Kale Salad	1 cup kale leaves chopped with 1 teaspoon honey and 1 tablespoon balsamic vinegar.
63	Chick Pea Salad	¼ chickpeas with 1 tablespoon sliced scallions, a squeeze of lemon juice, and ¼ cup diced tomatoes.
64	Grilled Garlic Corn on the Cob	: One small-sized ear brushed with 1 teaspoon sautéed minced garlic and 1 teaspoon olive oil, grilled until tender.
65	Pretzels & Cream Cheese	15 mini pretzel sticks with 2 tablespoons fat-free cream cheese.
66	Bacon Brussels Salad	Seven brussel spouts thinly sliced and mixed with one piece lean bacon, chopped.
67	Rosemary Potatoes	⅓ cup thinly sliced potato tossed with 1 teaspoons olive oil and a teaspoon of chopped rosemary.
68	Spicy Black	¼ cup black beans with 1

	Beans	tablespoon salsa and 1 tablespoon non-fat Greek yogurt.
69	Caprese Salad	1 ounce (hockey puck sized) of fresh mozzarella with ½ cup cherry tomatoes and 2 teaspoons of balsamic vinegar.
70	Goldfish	About 40 fishies...try the cheddar kind!
71	Chips n' Salsa	10 baked tortilla chips with ¼ cup salsa.
72	Mini Ham Sandwich	Two slices honey-baked ham with 2 teaspoons honey mustard rolled in a lettuce leaf.
73	Lox Bagel	½ whole-wheat mini bagel with two thin slices of lox.
74	Turkey Roll-Ups	Four slices smoked turkey rolled up and dipped in 2 teaspoons honey mustard.
75	Balsamic Veggies	3 cups raw peppers (any color!) dipped in 2 tablespoons balsamic reduction.

Sweet and Salty

76	Chocolate Trail Mix	Eight almonds, four chocolate chips, and 1 tablespoon raisins.
77	Apples and Cheese	1 non-fat mozzarella cheese stick with half of a baseball-sized apple (any variety), sliced.
78	PB & Celery	1 medium celery stalk with 1 tablespoon peanut butter.
79	Cottage Cheese Melon Boat	1 cup melon balls with ½ cup non-fat cottage cheese.

80	Carrot and Raisin Salad	1 cup shaved carrots with 2 tablespoons raisins and 1 tablespoon balsamic vinegar.
81	Tropical Cottage Cheese:	½ cup non-fat cottage cheese with ½ cup fresh mango and pineapple, chopped.
82	Blue-Cheese Stuffed Apricots	Three dried apricots with 1 tablespoon crumbled blue cheese.
83	Rice Cake and Almond Butter	One rice cake (try brown rice!) with 2 teaspoons almond butter.
84	Sweet n' Spicy Pecans	Five pecans roasted with 2 teaspoons maple syrup and 1 teaspoon cinnamon.
85	Apples n' Peanut Butter	½ an apple, sliced and dipped in 1 teaspoon natural peanut butter.
86	Chocolate Hazelnut Crackers	Four wheat thins dipped in 1 teaspoon Nutella (or other hazelnut spread).
87	Strawberry Salad	1 cup raw spinach with ½ cup sliced strawberries and 1 tablespoon balsamic.
88	Cacao-Roasted Almonds	Pop in eight almonds
89	Bell peppers	Delicious and crunchy one slice of bell pepper has just 2 calories!
90	Hummus	One of my fave go-to snacks. Packing just 23 calories per tablespoon, pair that with a 2

		calorie slice of bell pepper and you have a great under 50 calorie snack!
91	Strawberries	The perfectly sweet, but healthy snack has just 4 calories per berry.
92	Dill pickles	For only 8 calories per pickle, this snack will fulfill your crunch and salt craving in an instant.
93	Grapefruit	Great for a snack or breakfast, it has lots of vitamin C. For only 39 calories, you can have a half of one.
94	Popcorn	Not movie popcorn, but air popped and butter free, one whole cup has just 31 calories!
95	Cucumber	Seem like a funny snack? It's actually perfect for a hot day. Mostly made of water, you can nosh a whole cup of cucumber for only 14 calories.
96	Cantaloupe	This delicious fruit is full of fiber and has only 24 calories in an 1/8 of a melon.
97	Apricots	Juicy and filling, apricots are the perfect, 17 calorie addition to this list of 15 snacks under 50 calories.
98	Egg whites	At a mere 20 calories per white, eggs are filled with protein, which means a scrambled egg white will really keep you satisfied.
99	Olives	Filled with good fats, five olives have only 26 calories and are the

		perfect addition to a small salad.
100	Grapes	Packed with good-for-you things like antioxidants, 10 grapes are a great snack at only 35 calories.
101	Raisins	Sweet, chewy and delicious, one small packet of raisins is the ideal 42 calorie snack.
102	Kiwi fruit	Known also to improve sleep (yes, really!) one kiwi is a tart 47 calorie option.
103	Watermelon	My favorite summer fruit, a whole cup of watermelon is guilt free and refreshing on a hot day for just 48 calories.

Guilt-free snacking

104	Celery Sticks	Celery sticks just don't hit the spot, but these properly tasty low-calorie snacks will do the job
105	Apple	1 large apple and 5 almonds - 97 calories
106	Banana	1 small banana - 90 calories
107	Brussels Sprout	280g Brussels sprouts - 100 calories
108	Peaches	2 medium peaches - 76 calories
109	Blueberries	Punnet of blueberries and 1tbsp fat-free Greek yoghurt - 90 calories
110	Almonds	14 almonds - 98 calories
111	Figs	6 figs - 96 calories
112	Fruit salad	200g fruit salad - 82 calories
113	strawberry	1 pot of strawberry fromage frais and 6 cherries - 99 calories

114	Dried apricots	5 dried apricots - 95 calories
115	Dates	4 dates - 96 calories
116	Sweet potato	1 small sweet potato - 100 calories Once guilty pleasure
117	Pringles	10 Pringles - 100 calories
118	Strawberries	1 meringue nest with 6 strawberries - 100 calories
119	Gingerbread	1 mini gingerbread man - 80 calories
120	Jelly beans	25 Jelly Belly jelly beans - 100 calories
121	peanuts	Half a pint of lager and 7 peanuts - 99 calories Instant hit
122	Cereal bar	1 Kellogg's Fruit 'n Fibre cereal bar - 95 calories
123	Pitta	1 mini pitta bread with reduced-fat cottage cheese - 97 calories
124	Breaded ham	1 slice of breaded ham and 1tsp English mustard - 71 calories
125	oatcake	1 oatcake with 1tsp low-fat smooth peanut butter - 96 calories
126	crumpet	1 toasted crumpet and 1tsp low-fat grated cheese - 92 calories
127	fishfinger	1 fishfinger with 4tbsp reduced-sugar and salt baked beans - 91 calories
128	Tortilla wrap	1 Asda tortilla wrap - 97 calories
129	Frozen grapes	33 frozen grapes - 99 calories

130	Cheese	30g low-fat Edam cheese and 5 sticks of celery - 99 calories
131	Cream cheese	1tsp cream cheese on 1 plain Ryvita with 1 medium tomato - 100 calories
132	Cottage cheese	25g natural cottage cheese and 1 medium peach - 91 calories

Easy to make

133	Grilled bacon	1 rasher of grilled bacon and a dollop of ketchup - 87 calories
134	Brown toast	1 slice of brown toast and Marmite - 100 calories
135	Porridge oats	28g serving of porridge oats - 100 calories
136	Boiled egg	1 hard-boiled egg - 78 calories
137	Roasted chestnuts	5 roasted chestnuts - 100 calories
138	Rice cake	1 Dairylea slice and 1 rice cake - 99 calories
139	Cream crackers	2 cream crackers with 1tbsp reduced-fat coleslaw - 100 calories
140	Ryvitas	2 multigrain Ryvitas with Marmite - 83 calories
141	Boiled potato	1 sliced boiled potato with 1tbsp fresh salsa - 91 calories
142	breadsticks	4 breadsticks with tzatziki - 100 calories
143	Protein shake	28g Solgar Whey To Go protein shake - 100 calories
144	ham	2 slices of Parma ham with 6 thin slices of melon - 80 calories

145	Chicken soup	Heinz Weight Watchers Chicken Soup - 88 calories
146	yoghurt	1 Müller Light cherry yoghurt - 96 calories

Appendix D

Calorie contents of different foods

The following information has been collected from the web and is being provided for information purpose only.

Italian Food Calorie Content

Italian Food	Calories per typical serving
Starters	
Melon	40
Melon with Parma ham	150
Mozzarella and tomato salad (no dressing)	190
Mixed fish salad	220
Bruschetta	220
Minestrone soup	240
Tuna and bean salad	300
Garlic bread, 4 pieces	400
Main courses	
Spaghetti arrabiata	400
Mushroom risotto	475
Scampi provençale	500
Cannelloni	500
Ravioli	510

Chicken risotto	550
Spaghetti napoletana	630
Lasagne	650
Spaghetti marinara	690
Spaghetti bolognese	720
Pizza	750
Spaghetti carbonara	1,020
Desserts	
Gelati	140
Cassata	150
Zabaglione	185
Tiramisu	440

Greek Food Calorie Content

Greek Food	Calories per typical serving
Meze	
Olives, each	3
Tzatziki, 1 level tbsp	20
Melitzanosalata (aubergine purée salad), 1 level tbsp	30
Hummus, 1 level tbsp	40
Small portion of marinated calamari (squid)	50
Keftethes (meatballs), each	50
Taramasalata, 1 level tbsp	60
Pitta bread, 1/2 pitta	75
Starters	

Chicken soup and rice	100
Dolmades (stuffed vine leaves)	200
Marinated calamari	200
Main courses	
Greek salad without dressing	280
Baked fish with tomatoes and garlic	300
Lamb and pepper kebabs	320
Meatballs on skewers	445
Stifado (meat stew)	550
Meatballs	580
Moussaka	700
Spanakopitta (spinach and cheese pie)	700
Desserts	
Watermelon	30
Halva (sweetmeat made with honey and sesame seed)	260
Baklava (honey and walnut pastry)	320

Spanish Food Calorie Content

Spanish Food	Calories per typical serving
Tapas	
Setas alhomo (mushrooms in garlic sauce)	150
Pimiento relleno (stuffed pepper)	160
Arroz con pollo (rice with chicken)	200
Paella	200

Gambas al ajillo (garlic shrimp)	200
Mussels	220
Tortilla (Spanish omelette)	240
Calamari (deep fried squid)	250
Patatas bravas (fried potatoes in chilli and garlic sauce)	300
Boquerones (whitebait)	300
Lamb stew	350
Chorizo (spicy sausage)	400
Albondigas (meatballs in sauce)	400
Desserts	
Flan de almendras (almond flan)	270
Flan de leche (baked custard flan)	330
Arroz con leche (rice pudding)	400

Thai Food Calorie Content

Thai Food	**Calories per typical serving**
Starters	50
Fish cakes, each	100
Spring rolls, each	110
Gai tome ke (chicken, coconut and galangel soup)	120
Tom yam gung (hot and sour soup with prawns)	150
Yam talay (seafood salad) without dressing	400

Satay and peanut sauce	**Main courses**
Main courses	310
Moo pad king (pork fried with ginger)	370
Normai pad kai (pork with bamboo shoots)	400
Pla manow (fish with lemon sauce)	410
Pad Thai (fried noodles)	420
Gai hoh bai teo (chicken wrapped in bandan leaf)	540
Gang ped bhed yang (duck curry)	**Desserts**
Desserts	70
Fresh pineapple	210
Som loy geow (oranges in syrup)	665
Kow neuw mamuang (mangoes with sticky rice)	50

UK Food Calorie Content

UK Food	Calories per typical serving
Starters	
Melon	60
Tomato soup	150
Prawn cocktail	350
Breaded mushrooms with dip	370
Pâté and toast	400
Main courses	

Venison in red wine	280
Pork and apple casserole	360
Lancashire hotpot	400
Shepherd's pie	400
Fish pie	450
Beef casserole	490
225g/8oz well-done rump steak with chips	525
Roast beef with trimmings	540
225g/8oz well-done fillet steak and chips	550
Beef Wellington	560
Sausage and mash	585
Toad in the hole	640
Gammon steak and chips	680
Beef stew with dumplings	770
Scampi and chips	820
Steak and kidney pie with chips	820
Desserts	
Trifle	270
Lemon meringue pie	305
Spotted dick and custard	435
Apple pie and custard	435
Fruit crumble and custard	475
Treacle tart and custard	490
Cheesecake	495
Ice-cream sundae	500
Bread and butter pudding	505

| Sponge pudding and custard | 505 |
| Toad in the hole | 640 |

French Food Calorie Content

French Food	Calories per typical serving
Starters	
Mussels	190
Crudités with garlic mayonnaise	240
Grilled goat's cheese salad	240
Pâté de campagne	260
Snails	300
French onion soup	375
Shellfish bisque	500
Main courses	
Grilled Dover sole	220
Grilled trout	250
Chicken chasseur	480
Steak au poivre	490
Steak with béarnaise sauce	575
Moules mariniere with pommes frites	580
Coq au vin	585
Cassoulet	610
Beef bourguignon	635
Duck in orange sauce	840
Desserts	
Crème caramel	215

Chocolate mousse	250
Crème brûlée	350
Crêpe Suzette	400
Chocolate gateau	435
Tarte au citron	445
Tarte Tatin	525
Profiteroles	600

American and Mexican Food Calorie Content

American and Mexican Food	Calories per typical serving
Starters	
Barbecue ribs	360
Tortilla chips and salsa	515
Chicken wings with barbecue dip	520
Potato skins with sour cream	565
Tortilla chips and guacamole	590
Quesadilla	650
Nachos	1,000
Main courses	
Caesar salad	535
Chicken burrito	600
Chicken enchilada	615
Chicken chimichanga	675
Beef burritos	695
Beef enchilada	700
Beef chimichanga	765

Chilli cheeseburger and fries	775
Chilli con carne	800
Vegetable fajitas	810
350g/12oz well-done sirloin steak with fries	860
Chicken fajitas	1,035
Beef fajitas	1,300
Double cheeseburger with fries and coleslaw	2,120
Desserts	
Chocolate fudge cake	400
Banana split	400
Key lime pie with whipped cream	560
Mississippi mud pie	570
Pecan pie	690

Indian Food Calorie Content

Indian Food	**Calories per typical serving**
Starters	
Cucumber raita, 1tbsp	20
Tomato sambal, 1tbsp	20
Mango chutney, 1tbsp	60
Poppadom, each	65
Lime pickle, 1tbsp	70
Onion bhaji, each	190
Vegetable samosa, each	260
Meat samosa, each	320

Main courses	
Tandoori chicken	300
Aloo gobi	330
Vegetable curry	350
Keema madras	450
Aloo saag	500
Beef madras	540
Vegetable biriyani	550
Lamb bhuna	680
Chicken tikka masala	680
Chicken curry	700
Rogan josh	700
Chicken dhansk	720
Beef kheema	780
Chicken korma	870

Chinese Food Calorie Content

Chinese Food	Calories per typical serving
Starters	
Sesame prawn toasts, per piece	70
Hot and sour soup	80
Prawn wonton, each	80
Spare rib, each	140
Crab and sweetcorn soup	155
Chicken noodle soup	160
Chicken and sweetcorn soup	170

Crispy seaweed	200
Pancake roll	240
Main courses	
Chicken in lemon sauce	300
Chicken and pineapple	310
Beef in oyster sauce	340
Beef in yellow bean sauce	360
Beef with green peppers and black bean sauce	380
Chicken and cashew nuts	380
Chicken chop suey	425
Sweet and sour chicken	480
Crispy duck, four pancakes	800
Prawns balls (10) in batter with sweet and sour sauce	1,200

Source: http://www.weightlossresources.co.uk

Appendix E

Calorie burnt in exercises

In this appendix I'll share couple of tables from different sources that shows how much calorie you would burn based on your weight and activity. Both are collected from the web and are being shared only to help aspiring weight watchers to have a good understanding of calories burnt.

Exercise & Calories Burned per Hour	130 lbs	155 lbs	180 lbs	205 lbs
Aerobics, general	384	457	531	605
Aerobics, high impact	413	493	572	651
Aerobics, low impact	295	352	409	465
Aerobics, step aerobics	502	598	695	791
Archery	207	246	286	326
Backpacking, Hiking with pack	413	493	572	651
Badminton	266	317	368	419
Bagging grass, leaves	236	281	327	372
Bakery, light effort	148	176	204	233

Ballet, twist, jazz, tap	266	317	368	419
Ballroom dancing, fast	325	387	449	512
Ballroom dancing, slow	177	211	245	279
Basketball game, competitive	472	563	654	745
Basketball, playing, non game	354	422	490	558
Basketball, shooting baskets	266	317	368	419
Basketball, wheelchair	384	457	531	605
Bathing dog	207	246	286	326
Bird watching	148	176	204	233
Boating, power, speed boat	148	176	204	233
Bowling	177	211	245	279
Boxing, in ring	708	844	981	1117
Boxing, punching bag	354	422	490	558
Boxing, sparring	531	633	735	838
Calisthenics, light, pushups, situps...	207	246	286	326
Calisthenics, fast, pushups, situps...	472	563	654	745
Canoeing, camping trip	236	281	327	372
Canoeing, rowing, light	177	211	245	279
Canoeing, rowing, moderate	413	493	572	651
Canoeing, rowing, vigorous	708	844	981	1117
Carpentry, general	207	246	286	326
Carrying 16 to 24 lbs,	354	422	490	558

upstairs				
Carrying 25 to 49 lbs, upstairs	472	563	654	745
Carrying heavy loads	472	563	654	745
Carrying infant, level ground	207	246	286	326
Carrying infant, upstairs	295	352	409	465
Carrying moderate loads upstairs	472	563	654	745
Carrying small children	177	211	245	279
Children's games, hopscotch...	295	352	409	465
Circuit training, minimal rest	472	563	654	745
Cleaning gutters	295	352	409	465
Cleaning, dusting	148	176	204	233
Climbing hills, carrying up to 9 lbs	413	493	572	651
Climbing hills, carrying 10 to 20 lb	443	528	613	698
Climbing hills, carrying 21 to 42 lb	472	563	654	745
Climbing hills, carrying over 42 lb	531	633	735	838
Coaching: football, basketball, soccer	236	281	327	372
Coal mining, general	354	422	490	558
Construction, exterior, remodeling	325	387	449	512
Crew, sculling, rowing,	708	844	981	1117

competition				
Cricket (batting, bowling)	295	352	409	465
Croquet	148	176	204	233
Cross country snow skiing, slow	413	493	572	651
Cross country skiing, moderate	472	563	654	745
Cross country skiing, racing	826	985	1144	1303
Cross country skiing, uphill	974	1161	1348	1536
Cross country skiing, vigorous	531	633	735	838
Curling	236	281	327	372
Cycling, <10mph, leisure bicycling	236	281	327	372
Cycling, >20mph, racing	944	1126	1308	1489
Cycling, 10-11.9mph, light	354	422	490	558
Cycling, 12-13.9mph, moderate	472	563	654	745
Cycling, 14-15.9mph, vigorous	590	704	817	931
Cycling, 16-19mph, very fast, racing	708	844	981	1117
Cycling, mountain bike, bmx	502	598	695	791
Darts (wall or lawn)	148	176	204	233
Diving, springboard or platform	177	211	245	279
Downhill snow skiing,	354	422	490	558

moderate				
Downhill snow skiing, racing	472	563	654	745
Electrical work, plumbing	207	246	286	326
Farming, baling hay, cleaning barn	472	563	654	745
Farming, chasing cattle on horseback	236	281	327	372
Farming, feeding horses or cattle	266	317	368	419
Farming, feeding small animals	236	281	327	372
Farming, grooming animals	354	422	490	558
Fencing	354	422	490	558
Fire fighter, climbing ladder, full gear	649	774	899	1024
Fire fighter, hauling hoses on ground	472	563	654	745
Fishing from boat, sitting	148	176	204	233
Fishing from riverbank, standing	207	246	286	326
Fishing from riverbank, walking	236	281	327	372
Fishing in stream, in waders	354	422	490	558
Fishing, general	177	211	245	279
Fishing, ice fishing	118	141	163	186
Flying airplane (pilot)	118	141	163	186
Football or baseball,	148	176	204	233

playing catch				
Football, competitive	531	633	735	838
Football, touch, flag, general	472	563	654	745
Forestry, ax chopping, fast	1003	1196	1389	1582
Forestry, ax chopping, slow	295	352	409	465
Forestry, carrying logs	649	774	899	1024
Forestry, sawing by hand	413	493	572	651
Forestry, trimming trees	531	633	735	838
Frisbee playing, general	177	211	245	279
Frisbee, ultimate Frisbee	472	563	654	745
Gardening, general	236	281	327	372
General cleaning	207	246	286	326
Golf, driving range	177	211	245	279
Golf, general	266	317	368	419
Golf, miniature golf	177	211	245	279
Golf, using power cart	207	246	286	326
Golf, walking and pulling clubs	254	303	351	400
Golf, walking and carrying clubs	266	317	368	419

http://www.bodybuilding.com/fun/calories.htm

Calories burned in 30 minutes for people of three different weights

(This table was first printed in the July 2004 issue of the Harvard Heart Letter. For more information or to order, please go to http://www.health.harvard.edu/heart.)

The table below lists the calories burned by doing dozens of activities listed by category (such as gym activities, training and sports activities, home repair, etc.) for 30 minutes. In each category, activities are listed from least to most calories burned.

Gym Activities	125 pound person	155 pound person	185 pound person
Weight Lifting: general	90	112	133
Aerobics: water	120	149	178
Stretching, Hatha Yoga	120	149	178
Calisthenics: moderate	135	167	200
Riders: general (ie., HealthRider)	150	186	222
Aerobics: low impact	165	205	244
Stair Step Machine: general	180	223	266
Teaching aerobics	180	223	266
Weight Lifting:	180	223	266

vigorous			
Aerobics, Step: low impact	210	260	311
Aerobics: high impact	210	260	311
Bicycling, Stationery: moderate	210	260	311
Rowing, Stationery: moderate	210	260	311
Calisthenics: vigorous	240	298	355
Circuit Training: general	240	298	355
Rowing, Stationery: vigorous	255	316	377
Elliptical Trainer: general	270	335	400
Ski Machine: general	285	353	422
Aerobics, Step: high impact	300	372	444
Bicycling, Stationery: vigorous	315	391	466
Training and Sport Activities			
Billiards	75	93	111
Bowling	90	112	133
Dancing: slow, waltz, foxtrot	90	112	133
Frisbee	90	112	133

Volleyball: non-competitive, general play	90	112	133
Water Volleyball	90	112	133
Archery: non-hunting	105	130	155
Golf: using cart	105	130	155
Hang Gliding	105	130	155
Curling	120	149	178
Gymnastics: general	120	149	178
Horseback Riding: general	120	149	178
Tai Chi	120	149	178
Volleyball: competitive, gymnasium play	120	149	178
Walk: 3.5 mph (17 min/mi)	120	149	178
Badminton: general	135	167	200
Walk: 4 mph (15 min/mi)	135	167	200
Kayaking	150	186	222
Skateboarding	150	186	222
Snorkeling	150	186	222
Softball: general play	150	186	222
Walk: 4.5 mph (13 min/mi)	150	186	222
Whitewater: rafting, kayaking	150	186	222

Dancing: disco, ballroom, square	165	205	244
Golf: carrying clubs	165	205	244
Dancing: Fast, ballet, twist	180	223	266
Fencing	180	223	266
Hiking: cross-country	180	223	266
Skiing: downhill	180	223	266
Swimming: general	180	223	266
Walk/Jog: jog <10 min.	180	223	266
Water Skiing	180	223	266
Wrestling	180	223	266
Basketball: wheelchair	195	242	289
Race Walking	195	242	289
Ice Skating: general	210	260	311
Racquetball: casual, general	210	260	311
Rollerblade Skating	210	260	311
Scuba or skin diving	210	260	311
Sledding, luge, toboggan	210	260	311
Soccer: general	210	260	311
Tennis: general	210	260	311
Basketball: playing a game	240	298	355
Bicycling: 12-13.9 mph	240	298	355

Football: touch, flag, general	240	298	355
Hockey: field & ice	240	298	355
Rock Climbing: rappelling	240	298	355
Running: 5 mph (12 min/mile)	240	298	355
Running: pushing wheelchair, marathon wheeling	240	298	355
Skiing: cross-country	240	298	355
Snow Shoeing	240	298	355
Swimming: backstroke	240	298	355
Volleyball: beach	240	298	355
Bicycling: BMX or mountain	255	316	377
Boxing: sparring	270	335	400
Football: competitive	270	335	400
Orienteering	270	335	400
Running: 5.2 mph (11.5 min/mile)	270	335	400
Running: cross-country	270	335	400
Bicycling: 14-15.9 mph	300	372	444
Martial Arts: judo, karate, kick box	300	372	444
Racquetball:	300	372	444

competitive			
Rope Jumping	300	372	444
Running: 6 mph (10 min/mile)	300	372	444
Swimming: breaststroke	300	372	444
Swimming: laps, vigorous	300	372	444
Swimming: treading, vigorous	300	372	444
Water Polo	300	372	444
Rock Climbing: ascending	330	409	488
Running: 6.7 mph (9 min/mile)	330	409	488
Swimming: butterfly	330	409	488
Swimming: crawl	330	409	488
Bicycling: 16-19 mph	360	446	533
Handball: general	360	446	533
Running: 7.5 mph (8 min/mile)	375	465	555
Running: 8.6 mph (7 min/mile)	435	539	644
Bicycling: > 20 mph	495	614	733
Running: 10 mph (6 min/mile)	495	614	733
Outdoor Activities			
Planting seedlings, shrubs	120	149	178

Raking Lawn	120	149	178
Sacking grass or leaves	120	149	178
Gardening: general	135	167	200
Mowing Lawn: push, power	135	167	200
Operate Snow Blower: walking	135	167	200
Plant trees	135	167	200
Gardening: weeding	139	172	205
Carrying & stacking wood	150	186	222
Digging, spading dirt	150	186	222
Laying sod / crushed rock	150	186	222
Mowing Lawn: push, hand	165	205	244
Chopping & splitting wood	180	223	266
Shoveling Snow: by hand	180	223	266
Home & Daily Life Activities			
Sleeping	19	23	28
Watching TV	23	28	33
Reading: sitting	34	42	50
Standing in line	38	47	56
Cooking	75	93	111
Child-care: bathing,	105	130	155

feeding, etc.			
Food Shopping: with cart	105	130	155
Moving: unpacking	105	130	155
Playing w/kids: moderate effort	120	149	178
Heavy Cleaning: wash car, windows	135	167	200
Child games: hop-scotch, jacks, etc.	150	186	222
Playing w/kids: vigorous effort	150	186	222
Moving: household furniture	180	223	266
Moving: carrying boxes	210	260	311
Home Repair			
Auto Repair	90	112	133
Wiring and Plumbing	90	112	133
Carpentry: refinish furniture	135	167	200
Lay or remove carpet/tile	135	167	200
Paint, paper, remodel: inside	135	167	200
Cleaning rain gutters	150	186	222
Hanging storm windows	150	186	222

Paint house: outside	150	186	222
Carpentry: outside	180	223	266
Roofing	180	223	266
Occupational Activities			
Computer Work	41	51	61
Light Office Work	45	56	67
Sitting in Meetings	49	60	72
Desk Work	53	65	78
Sitting in Class	53	65	78
Truck Driving: sitting	60	74	89
Bartending/Server	75	93	111
Heavy Equip. Operator	75	93	111
Police Officer	75	93	111
Theater Work	90	112	133
Welding	90	112	133
Carpentry Work	105	130	155
Coaching Sports	120	149	178
Masseur, standing	120	149	178
Construction, general	165	205	244
Coal Mining	180	223	266
Horse Grooming	180	223	266
Masonry	210	260	311
Forestry, general	240	298	355
Heavy Tools, not power	240	298	355

| Steel Mill: general | 240 | 298 | 355 |
| Firefighting | 360 | 446 | 533 |

Appendix F

Atkin's Diet

The Atkins diet is a type of diet that promotes low carbohydrate and more protein rich diet. It was proposed and popularized by Dr. Robert Atkins.

The basic idea of this type of dieting is simple: make the body burn stored fat to create energy than to use glucose. This process is called *ketosis* which is triggered with low insulin levels, mostly before eating. Low level of insulin induces *lipolysis* which consumes fat to produce ketone bodies.

Dr Atkins' tried to establish that low-carbohydrate diet provides some advantage regarding metabolism as burning fat takes more calories. He estimated this advantage to be 950 calories per day. However a review study published in *Lancet* concluded that there was no such metabolic advantage. The reason why it might have been working was more due to the fact that people simply ate less as the diet offered little varieties and could get pretty boring.

To elaborate:

Sugars and starches like potatoes, rice, and bread are replaced with protein and fat like chicken, meat, and eggs. How it works? A carb-heavy meal floods the blood with glucose, too much for the cells to use. This extra energy is stored and eventually gets converted into fat.

Does it help to lose weight?

Yes, initial first few weeks it does seem to reduce some weight. However, it has no long term effect on weight and may actually cause the participants heartache when they notice no matter how hard they follow they simply do not lose any more weight.

In addition there are other problems. There are no solid, long term studies of this type of dieting to suggest that it would be beneficial for the body when it comes to diabetes and cholesterol, blood pressure, reducing the risk of heart attack. Actually, the extra amount of fat that is absorbed in the body may actually have some negative impact.

But, it should also be mentioned here while there are no solid benefit there are no serious bad effect as well. It is possible that some people may suffer from weakness, nausea, dizziness, constipation, irritability, and bad breath. If it has any long term effect that is not known as there are no such study to support that.

Some other details:

Atkin's diet allows high fat diet, almost in the range of 60%. Generally this is recommended to be within 30% of daily required calories. It recommends usual amount of protein but do not provide any suggestion on Carbohydrates.

As far as salt, Fiber, Potassium, Calcium, Vitamin B-12, D are considered Atkin's diet generally provides essential amount, perhaps little more on the sodium.

How difficult to follow?

Most of us are used to high carbohydrate diet. Moving away from it for protein and fat rich meat products are not that easy. Still, people can get used to it and continue to do it for months after months. But, as it is easily understood the varieties are much less and food may become boring after few days.

Studies has been conducted to find out if people following Atkin's diet had a higher rate of fall out than normal dieters. It did show higher percentages of Atkins dieters dropping out at 3, 6, 12, and 24 months than others did on a low-fat diet, but the differences were not significant. Two other studies that included low-carb dieters concluded diet type wasn't connected to dropout rate.

Fullness:

Filling full is an important thing in any diet. It scores good in that area as Protein and fat generally take longer than carbs to digest; this means we won't be feeling hungry too soon after eating a meal that is rich on meat.

Taste:

While burgers and cheese are very delicious and well loved eating them without the essential buns is bound to become a problem at some point.

It should be mentioned here that the U.S. government's Dietary Guidelines do not recommend Atkin's as its high fat diet directly contradicts low-fat diet that it touts.

It should also be mentioned that Atkins do not restrict vegetables. Throughout the plan, the dieter can eat more vegetables on a daily basis than is recommended by USDA guidelines. One can easily avoid almost all saturated fats on Atkins by following the plan as a vegetarian.

www.ingramcontent.com/pod-product-compliance
Lightning Source LLC
Chambersburg PA
CBHW050117280326
41933CB00010B/1144